DressYourBest

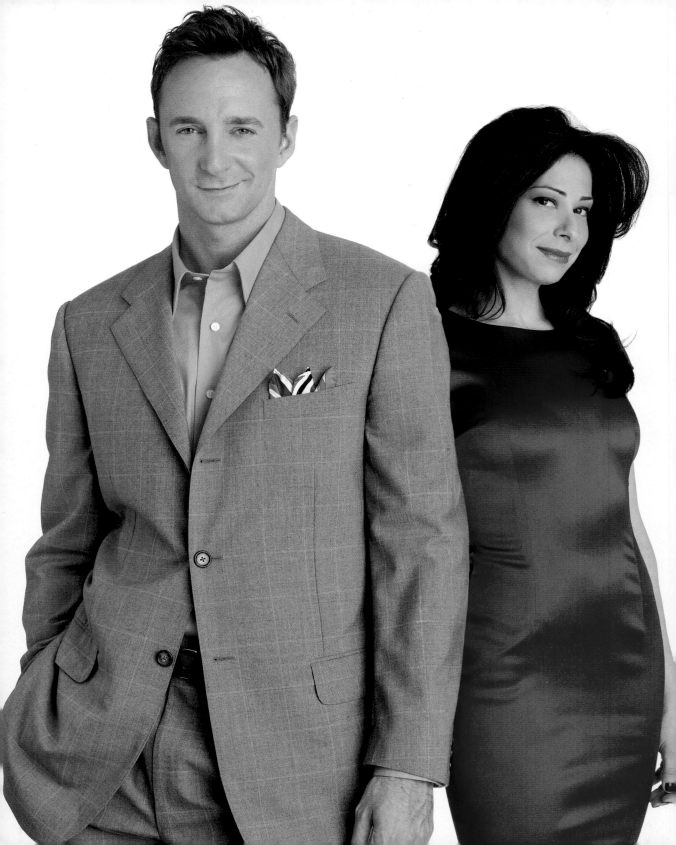

DressYourBest

The Complete Guide to Finding
the Style That's Right for Your Body

Clinton Kelly and Stacy London

Three Rivers Press, New York

Photographer: Brian Doben
Production manager: Nancy Corbett
Project manager: Christa Bourg
Casting: Alonna Friedman
Market editors: Eileen Goh, Lee Harper, Jessica Neff, Kimberly Suggs
Fashion assistants: Jeriana Hochberg, Garrett Munce, Deirdre Wegner, Lindsay ("Ashley") Weiner
Hair: Regee Drummer
Makeup: Deanna Nickel, Matthew Nigara
Photo assistants: Steve ("The Wizard") Giralt, Brad DeCecco, Masa Noguchi, Yoshi Suito
Catering: Ania Jozwik

Published in the United States by Three Rivers Press, an imprint of the Crown Publishing Group,
a division of Random House, Inc., New York.
www.crownpublishing.com

THREE RIVERS PRESS and the Tugboat design are registered trademarks of Random House, Inc.

Library of Congress Cataloging-in-Publication Data
Kelly, Clinton, and Stacy London.
Dress your best: the complete guide to finding the style that's right for your body / Clinton Kelly
and Stacy London.—1st ed. 1. Clothing and dress—Psychological aspects. 2. Fashion—
Psychological aspects. I. London, Stacy. II. Title.
GT524.K45 2005
391—dc22   2005013681

ISBN 0-307-23671-4

Printed in the United States of America

Design by Elizabeth Van Itallie

10 9 8 7 6 5 4 3

First Edition

This book is dedicated to anyone
who has ever looked into a full-length mirror
and thought, "It's hopeless."

It's not! We promise.

Contents

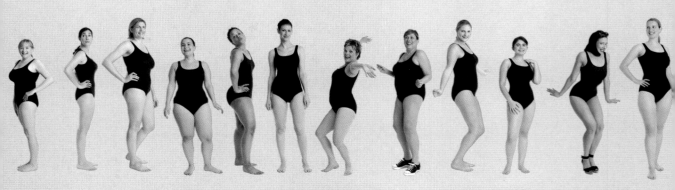

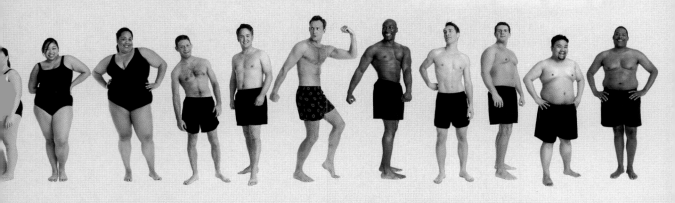

Introduction

We know what you're going through. We really do.

We realize clothes shopping can be hard work. Finding and maintaining your personal style can be exhausting. Finding anything that fits is enough to send you running for those "comfortable" sweatpants. Well, you can relax. Well, maybe not *relax*. We want you to use this book and make it work for you. Perhaps it might be better to say that we want your shopping experience to be a more pleasant one and your wardrobe to be better fitting.

Shopping off the rack is an exercise in frustration. Part of what makes us unique is what makes standardized sizing so difficult—we come in all different shapes and sizes. And not all those permutations are represented by a number on a size label. But recognizing this fact and accepting it is the first step in learning to make your clothes work for your body instead of feeling like it's your body that doesn't fit.

We set out to make this book a primer, a guide to the variety of body types and the kinds of clothes that suit them best.

Of course we couldn't show every conceivable body type, but we've done our best to show as many as possible. Now might be a good time for us to thank our very brave models—real people willing to be photographed in bathing suits in hopes that you could identify with their physiques and apply the lessons learned. And just to make things fair, we stripped down, too. And we thank you for buying this book so we can pay our therapists for helping us deal with the trauma.

A Word About Proportion

We've all heard that balance is the key to a happy life—work a little, play a little, relax a little. Well, the same principle applies to dressing as well. The key to looking your best is creating a balanced body shape through clothing. For example, if you're a little bit bigger on the bottom than you are on the top, there are ways to add a little extra emphasis to your upper body and make your entire frame proportionate. You'll see how this is done in the pages to come.

We often look to America's favorite couple when it comes to an "ideal" body proportion. Who might that couple be, you ask. No, not Brad Pitt and Jennifer Aniston. It's Barbie and Ken. Yes, two plastic dolls whose breakup was heard 'round the world, just like Brad and Jen's.

Now, don't misunderstand us. We're not saying that blond hair and big boobs are ideal for women, nor that rock-hard abs are essential for a man. Rather, we're talking about the genius of their proportions. Think of Barbie's short torso, long legs, small waist, and curvy hips. And picture Ken's broad shoulders and narrow waist. These are the proportions you can achieve with a little bit of effort.

Determining Your Current Body Shape

This is not rocket science. You don't even need a tape measure. Just stand in front of a full-length mirror in your underwear, scary as that may sound, and take a look at yourself. (Stacy had a Jack Daniels on the rocks and Clinton had a Tanqueray and tonic before attempting this exercise. Worked like a charm!)

Take a look at your body's proportion. Women, scrutinize shoulders, chest, waistline, hips, and overall height. And don't forget to turn around and check out your tush while you're at it. Men, see how your shoulders relate to your waistline and where you carry the bulk of your weight, if anywhere, and of course, take note of your height.

Then, think about how your clothes fit on the various parts of your body. Just because you can get a pair of pants on and fasten the button does not mean they fit. You have to be able to breathe, move without pain, and above all, sit down. If pants fit you in the hip, are they too tight at the waist? Chances are you have a little extra in the middle. Do you have problems finding jackets and shirts that fit you in the shoulder but not in the chest? You're curvy on top. Do your pants gape at the waistline when they fit in the hip? You're curvy on bottom. Is it impossible for you to find tailored clothing that doesn't drown your frame? You're most likely not curvy. Being able to isolate the area that gives you the most angst in the dressing room will aid you in figuring out which body type section in this book may apply to you.

Now, How to Use This Book

You may find your body is closest to one type, but chances are you will find tips in other sections that also apply. There are a finite number of clothing shapes. Different body types can wear the same shape for different effects. So you'll see how a curvy girl can wear a pencil skirt to accent her curves *and* how a not-so-curvy girl can wear one to create those curves. Keep in mind that it is just as important to read about body types which you think don't apply to you, so you can understand why certain looks work better on some people than on others.

The looks we've presented are *concepts,* not *ultimatums.* There will always be lots of options in terms of the types of clothes each body type can wear. We made our choices based on what was available in the market, and you'll have to do the same.

For example, on page 80 Bette is wearing a three-quarter-length tweed coat. If you live in Miami and you're reading this in July, we don't recommend you go out and buy a tweed coat, unless you enjoy heatstroke. But if you do relate to Bette's build, it's the *shape* of the coat that matters most, so go out and find a coat with the same proportion in a more climate-appropriate material.

We've also included a mini-glossary to help you with some terminology we've used throughout the book that you might not be familiar with—from *schweaters* to *shantung.*

Some Assorted Stuff We Feel Strongly About

Dress your body the way it is now. Do not wait until you "lose that last 10 pounds" or "bench press 350" to use this book. Because while we don't want to discourage you from your goals, our goal is to dress you in the present. What we've learned is that looking good *now* will help you feel better later. Walking around in oversized sweats makes you look like you've given up. And you may start to internalize that feeling. So, this is one time in life when a quick fix can actually have long-term effects. We've seen it hundreds of times. Don't wait for what may or may not change about you in the future. You are perfect now. So read this book and get shopping.

Tapered jeans. With all of our research, we have yet to find one person whose body has been flattered by wearing a tapered jean. While we're still trying to unravel the mystery involving the continuous sale of this item, we hereby declare a boycott of this style. If you own a pair, just burn 'em. And perhaps the manufacturers will take note.

Tailoring. Get used to the idea that everyone, regardless of body shape, can benefit from some alteration to their clothes once in a while. High-end stores usually offer complimentary alteration service. But for the rest of us, tailoring clothes to fit perfectly, regardless of price point, will make them look infinitely more expensive. We've found that women are willing to settle for a fit that's "close enough" when buying clothes off the rack, while men hardly ever buy a suit without its being fit to their bodies. So women, get those hemlines off the ground, pull in your waistline, make your sleeves shorter, and keep a seamstress in business. For a nominal fee, the clothes you own will no longer be "close enough"; the fit will be fabulous.

Quality over quantity any day. In America we've taken to buying in bulk—from toothpaste to tuna fish, paper towels to peanut butter. And unfortunately we do the same with our clothes. Instead of buying five sweatshirts at thirty bucks apiece, buy one cashmere sweater that fits you wonderfully. So what if you wear it to the office a couple of times a week. Your coworkers aren't keeping track of your wardrobe. And if they are, they should be fired because they're not paying enough attention to their jobs. What matters is that you look good in your clothes, not that you have seven different-colored sweatshirts for every day of the week.

So, Enough Talk

Now that we've outlined some of our ground rules and explained a few dos and don'ts, it's time to see these principles put to work. Turn the page and let's get going.

All Our Best (and Dress Your Best!),

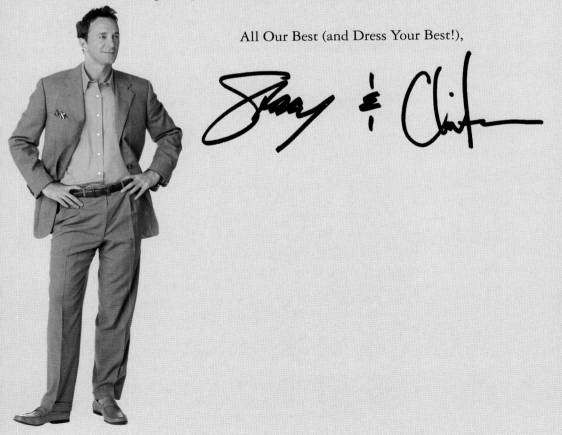

The Women

Essentials for Every Woman

- A black pantsuit
- A softer neutral suit with pants or skirt (gray, brown, khaki, or navy)
- 3 pairs of neutral trousers
- 3 winter-weight skirts (1 should be a tweed)
- 3 summer-weight skirts (1 should be a tweed)
- 3 cotton button-front shirts
- 3 blouses
- 2 sparkly tops
- Leather jacket
- Denim jacket
- Trench coat
- 3 pairs of jeans (all hemmed to different lengths, for flats, heels, and sandals)

- Black dress
- Solid-color dress
- Print or embellished dress
- 6 sweaters (3 neutral, 3 color, and vary necklines: crew, V-neck, and cardigan)
- 3 blazers (1 summer weight, 1 three-season weight, 1 winter weight)
- ¾-length wool coat
- Watch with 2 bands (leather and link)
- Black bag
- Brown bag
- Color or print bag
- Black heels
- Brown heels
- Color or print or embellished heels
- Black boots
- Brown boots
- Black flats

(To be honest, you can never have enough bags or shoes. They pop the most boring clothes into the next season and always keep things fresh . . . but we're talking *essentials* here.)

Bigger on Top, Overall

DON'T accentuate the narrowness of your lower half by wearing very narrow trousers or skirts—you just create even more disproportion between your top and bottom halves, making your chest look bigger.

DO create an overall streamlined look by adding a bit of volume (not bulk) to your lower half.

MUST-HAVES: The best bra you can afford. And an A-line skirt that falls below the knee. Yes, all heights need this length to balance out a larger chest.

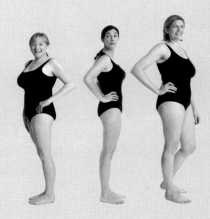

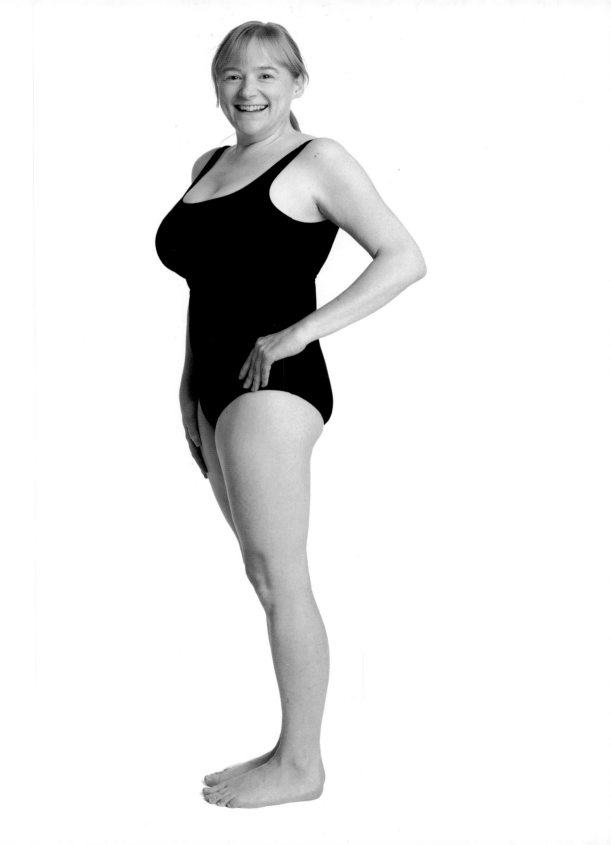

Bigger on Top,
Petite

CLARE
5-foot-2
Size 12 on top
Size 6 on bottom

"My chest is the bane of my existence. I know some people think it's great to have big boobs, but, honestly, my top half is so much bigger than my bottom half, it can be overwhelming. I normally wear sweaters with T-shirts underneath to disguise the size of my chest a little and cords or jeans. There just doesn't seem to be lots to do with a body shape like mine."

STACY AND CLINTON SAY: "*Au contraire,* Clare. There's lots you can do with a body shape like yours. While a top-heavy body can be the most difficult type to balance, it isn't impossible. Having a larger chest can, unfortunately, trick the eye and make you appear heavier than you actually are. So, first of all, if you have big 'girls,' take care of them. Get professionally fitted for your bras and buy as many different styles of them as you can afford. Second, you need structure! The more structured the clothes, the more effectively they'll change the shape of the body itself. The drapier the clothing, the more work your body has to do: the clothes just lie there. And the only way to get a longer, leaner line on this body type is to add volume—not bulk—to the bottom half."

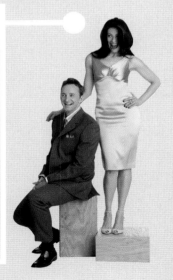

A Word About Hosiery

Opaque tights and hose work best for day. Sheer works best for evening. Never ever wear seamed toe (or worse, reinforced seamed toe) with an open-toe shoe. It's like wearing a white athletic sock with a sandal. Also, pay attention to the "denier" of hose. The denier is the number which describes the degree of opacity in the hose. The lower the number, the sheerer the hose, and the higher the number, the more opaque. In the United States, we have taken to wearing hose in the mid-denier range—the pseudo-sheer, if you will. Unfortunately, nothing matronizes an outfit more. Just add sneakers and we're back in the days of Melanie Griffith in *Working Girl*.

Bigger on Top,
Petite
Work

Multibutton jackets aren't the *only* ones that work for busty women. A one-button jacket with a high stance (button hits directly below bustline) cinches at the smallest part of the torso, supports the bustline, and visually gives a higher curve to the torso than a lower-stance jacket would.

While we never want petites in anything too long, the line of this jacket intentionally falls over the top of the hip to add width to the hip.

Jackets with straight placket pockets on top of the hip create volume at the hip and focus attention away from the chest.

Whatever underpinning you choose for the jacket, make sure to leave some skin showing up by the face and to wear a supportive **bra** underneath.

A softly draped A-line skirt serves to balance out the top half. Any straight or narrow skirt would simply serve to emphasize the difference between Clare's upper and lower halves. A stiffer construction, like a knife-pleated skirt, would add bulk and create an even larger, bulkier silhouette, but a softer A-line creates balancing volume to Clare's lower half, which is still flattering to her overall body shape.

Usually we advise petites to keep their skirts above the knee, but when you're petite with a larger chest, the skirt should cover the kneecap. The extra length in the skirt is needed to balance the size of the chest. Any shorter and you'll look top-heavy.

If we give Clare a closed-toe pointy shoe instead of a peep-toe, she could easily wear hosiery here. We want to balance her top half without shortening her leg. A small-textured tight, like a herringbone, in a slightly lighter shade than her suit, will create a professional look without making her legs look heavy.

Universal Tip: If you gain or lose 10 pounds, make sure to get refitted for your bras! Your size can change significantly with weight fluctuation.

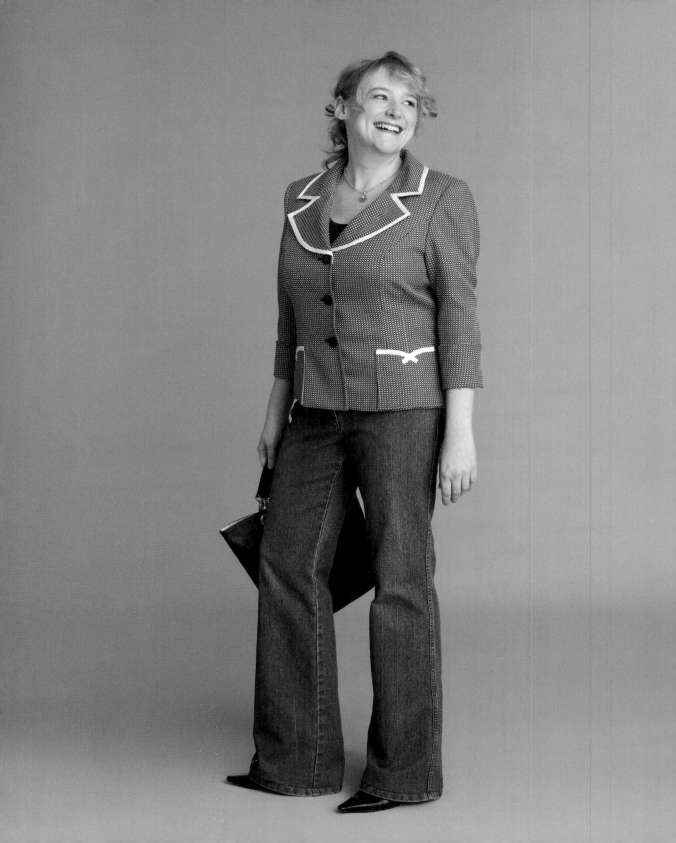

Bigger on Top,
Petite
Weekend

A favorite piece of ours for larger chests is the three-button jacket. It locks and loads the chest in and up, and stops it from spreading outward into arm territory. (A good bra will do this as well.) A narrower silhouette is created by a visual distinction between the arm and the torso.

Look for jackets with distracting visual interest. Here, the notched lapel with contrast **piping** draws attention away from the chest area.

The three-quarter sleeve further distinguishes the arm from the torso.

This jacket has a straighter, slightly boxier construction, but it still minimizes the bust and doesn't narrow at the bottom, which creates one straight line down from the chest to the top of the hip.

A wide-leg jean adds the volume necessary to balance a large chest without being exaggerated. But be careful, it's easy to slip into a baggy, unstructured, "painter pant" jean here and that is not what we want. Anything too wide is going to give you a dumpy butt.

Stick with a slightly lighter wash on the jeans than you might usually go for to balance a chest. A lighter wash is more noticeable as it reflects light and maximizes the focus on the leg.

And yes, a pointy boot keeps the outfit long and lean, but the shoes also look polished and stop the jean from looking sloppy. The jean has been intentionally left slightly long to balance the top half of the body. (It's the same theory as leaving the skirt longer in the previous look and in the next.)

Universal Tip: Contrast piping in small doses can pull focus away from problem areas, but too much of it, and you start to look like you're starring in a Shirley Temple movie. Mix and match it with denim or another casual fabric to keep it fresh.

I think I ate about a dozen olives while shooting this picture. Even though we were drinking martinis, we love the color cognac for evening. A nice way to stand out—it's not black, but not bright either.

Bigger on Top,
Petite
Evening

For evening, you might want to play up the chest a little bit. This style of dress is ideal because it displays some cleavage while supporting the breast line.

The seaming distinguishes the chest and the waist and adds a subtle A-line flare to the hip, bringing the entire body into balance.

Look for straps thick enough to **conceal** a supportive bra.

When you have a large chest, you can lose your midsection and look heavier. Make sure to find dresses that nip in at the waistline. Here the horizontal ruching at the waist clearly defines the waist and adds a more hourglass effect.

Because the vertical pleating on the breast is tightly sewn flat, it does not add volume to the chest.

Always look for a flattering neckline. Show skin around the neck and décolleté to lengthen the neck and add some proportion to the chest.

Look for soft folds in the skirt of a dress like this to balance the top half without adding conspicuous volume.

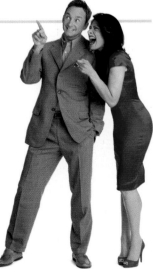

Universal Tip: While we have said that we don't like bra straps showing, if you've got a sexy lacy evening bra, it is okay to expose a little of the trim, just the way you might with a camisole under a V-neck sweater.

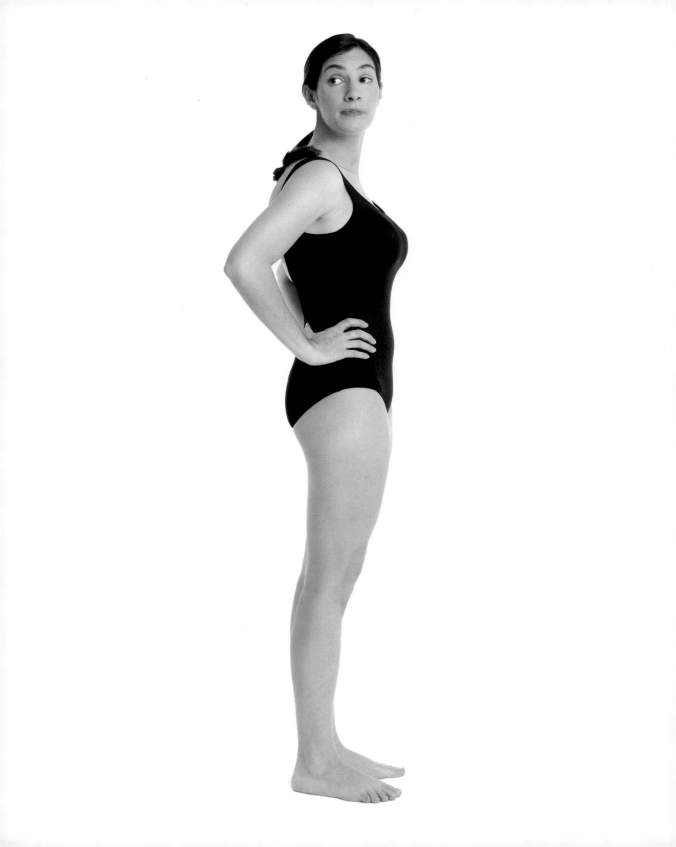

Bigger on Top,
Average Height

LAUREN
5-foot-5
Size 6 on top
Size 4 on bottom

"I'm big on top, but much smaller in the middle. That makes it impossible to buy tops and dresses. Anything that fits my chest is way too big in the middle and makes me look like I weigh more than I do. Things that work for my waist are way too tight in the chest and then I'm a 'sweater girl,' as my grandmother would say. It's tough being out of proportion. I know there might be other women who wouldn't mind my problem, but I've always been the 'serious' type. I wanted guys and other people to notice me for my mind, not my chest. That's why I spent years hiding it. I don't want to hide anymore, but I'm not prepared to flaunt it. I need help finding the middle ground."

STACY AND CLINTON SAY: "You say 'sweater girl' like it's a bad thing. Hello, Doris Day! But we understand not wanting to feel like you're out of balance. When the chest is slightly larger than your hips, there are subtle tricks that can bring the body back into alignment."

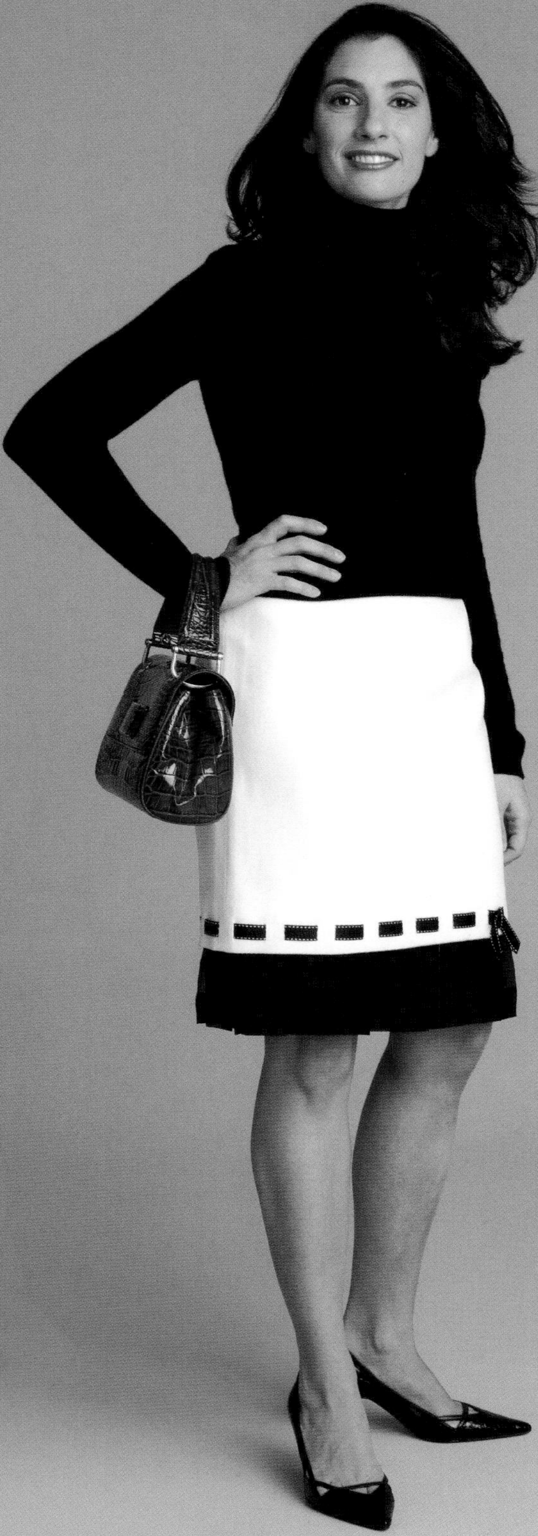

We'll let you in
on a little secret: this
white skirt is actually
a white dress, but we
loved it and topped it
with a sweater to cre-
ate the effect on
Lauren's body we
were looking for. You
can do the same!

Bigger on Top,
Average Height

Work

We love black and white for day. It is eternally classic. Think *My Fair Lady.*

Try doing a darker color on your top half and a lighter color on the bottom to pull a bit more focus away from the chest line. (Reverse this idea if you are slightly bigger on the bottom—works both ways!) Remember: Darker clothes camouflage, lighter colors emphasize, but *fit* is everything.

Up top, choose knits that keep a close line on the body. They complement without exaggerating the body frame.

Try straight skirts to emphasize hip and thigh and to balance the upper half. At an average height, skirts should just about cover the knee.

Look for features that reemphasize and frame the hip and upper-thigh area, like the same or similar color trim as the top.

Ahhh, the turtleneck. Clean. Classic. As long as you don't actually look like a turtle in it. Lauren has a thin neck and thin limbs. By selecting a dark turtleneck for her, we can emphasize the smallness of her frame *and* deemphasize a larger chest at the same time

Universal Tip: You don't have to match your bag to your shoes! And on a black-and-white outfit, do one accessory that really pops to make a statement.

Universal Tip: A pointy-toe shoe with a kitten heel is ideal for work with any skirt silhouette. It's flattering to the leg and comfortable to wear! *Honest!*

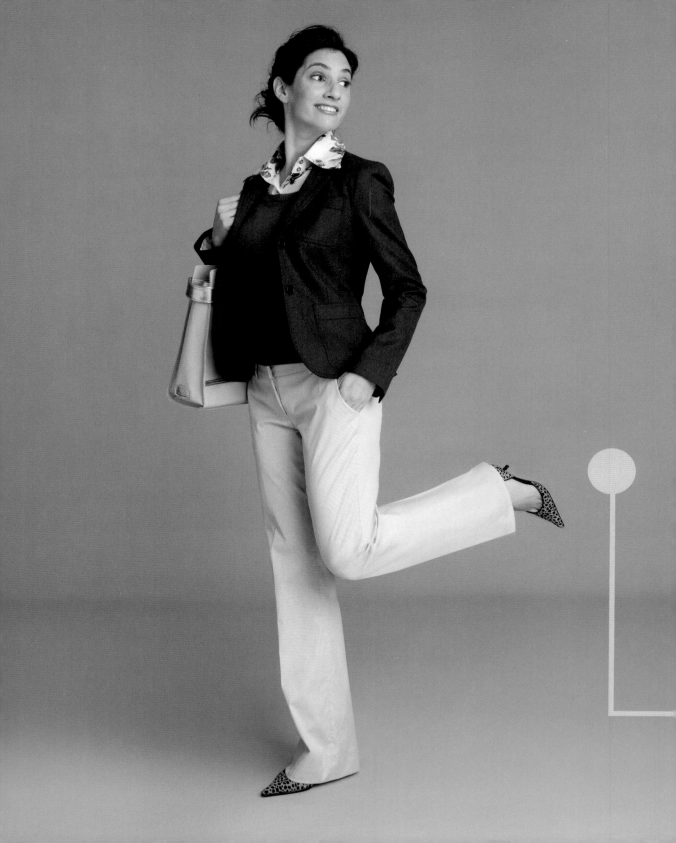

Bigger on Top,
Average Height
Weekend

Look for fitted, short boxy jackets with two or three buttons for the lock-and-load effect. In other words, they keep the chest in the middle of the torso instead of letting The Girls roam past the line of the arm.

Go for a narrow lapel on a jacket to call less attention to the chest area.

Look for a well-fit and snug shoulder to decrease the overall frame of the torso.

High armholes on jackets mean thinner sleeve widths. Stick to them to create distinction between the arm and the chest.

We love schweaters! That's a sweater with a built-in shirt collar and cuff. It adds visual interest and depth to an outfit without actually having to layer pieces and add bulk. There is a great range of these items in the marketplace. Look for ones that have detachable collars and cuffs to change the look up.

Don't go for too skinny a pant in the width of the leg. You'll throw the body out of proportion—your top half will only look bigger if you emphasize a narrow hip.

On bottom, try lighter colors, which will look wider than darker ones. It's about adding volume by tricking the eye without adding actual bulk.

A word of caution about khakis: don't do a pant that is too similar to your skin tone. If you have darker or olive skin, look for some with a lighter yellow undertone. If you have lots of pink in your skin, look for khakis with a bluish undertone. Nothing looks worse than a pant that exactly matches your flesh.

Universal Tip: Don't be afraid to mix patterns like florals and animal prints, but don't let either overpower an outfit. Use them as you would use spices in your favorite dish—as accents and sparingly!

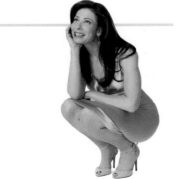

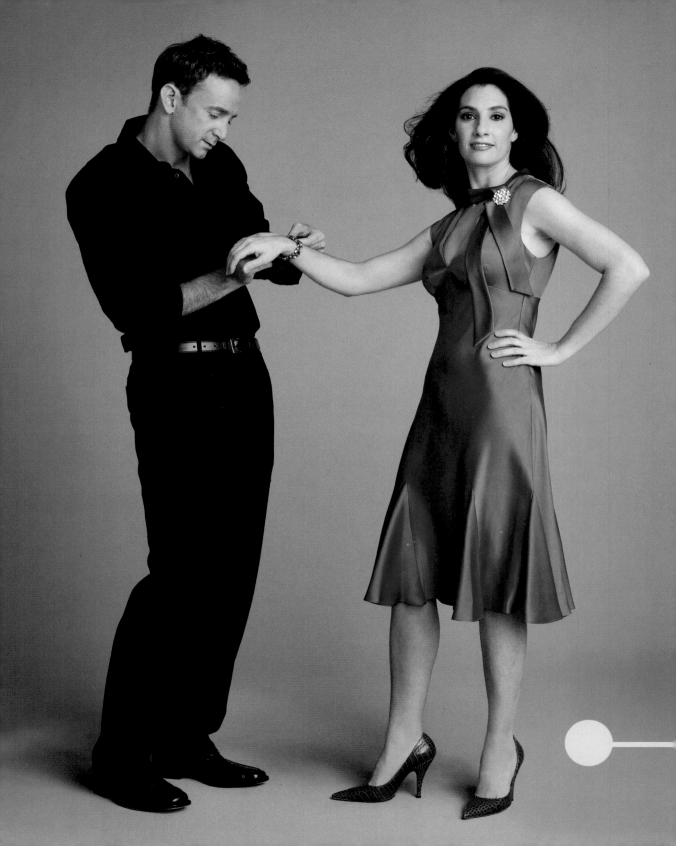

Bigger on Top,
Average Height
Evening

We loved this dress on Lauren. It just looked so classic yet modern, and really worked on her body type at the same time.

Brunettes with brown eyes don't seem to wear blues all that much. What, did we miss the memo saying the color was reserved for people with blue eyes? Lauren reminded us that we should tell more brown-eyed girls to wear blues.

Look for dresses that have an empire seam, which supports the **bustline** and raises the eye line above the natural waist, creating length in the body overall.

The top half of the dress is cut to cover a supportive bra. Please, ladies, if you have a larger chest, do not attempt dresses that would require you to go braless. There are plenty of sexy deep-V–cut dresses, and deep plunge bras to go with them, so that you don't delve into the world of spaghetti straps and halter tops . . . or God forbid, backless tops.

Try dresses that are narrow in the hip and cut on the bias. Such cuts emphasize the hip and keep it in proportion with the bust.

A soft A-line with inverted pleats balances the proportion of the whole body: between the shoulder, chest, hip, and leg.

This particular dress, while having a pretty deep V, also had a scarf tie. This is an optional feature to deemphasize the chest. We liked pinning it to the side with a brooch, but again, this is a decorative, not functional, aspect of the dress.

Universal Tip: Crocodile shoes, whether real or embossed leather, are usually reserved for day wear, but you can also do them for evening—especially if they're in a great color that happens to go perfectly with the color of your dress.

Universal Tip: With deep-V dresses, busty women now have options when it comes to bras; clear front straps allow for bust support without everyone knowing it.

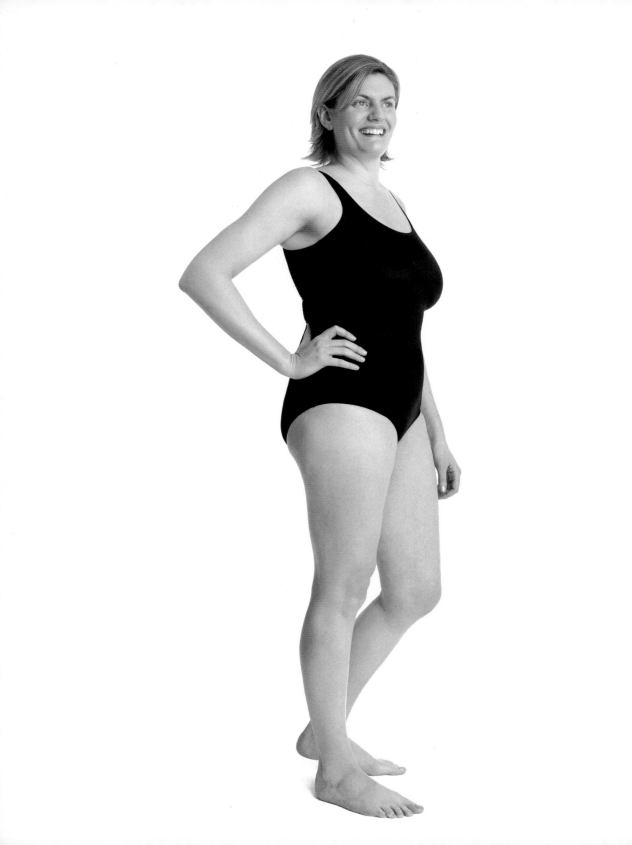

Bigger on Top,
Tall

MEREDITH
5-foot-11
Size 16 on top
Size 12 on bottom

"Since I was quite young, I have been very tall. It was tough in the awkward teen years, when I would wear only flats and do everything I could to appear shorter, but now I am genuinely happy to be tall. That said, being five-eleven does present certain wardrobe challenges. For one, nearly every pair of pants and every shirt that I buy needs to be let down in the hem and sleeves or else I appear to have outgrown my clothes (not a good look!). To make matters more interesting, most of my height is in my legs and I have a larger-than-average chest. Sometimes shopping for clothes can be frustrating because it seems that the latest styles are designed for petite women with no chest."

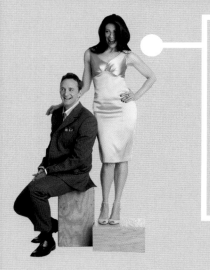

STACY AND CLINTON SAY: "Some saying comes to mind about green grass and a fence. We all have our issues to contend with when it comes to dressing our bodies. What's stunning about your body type is that you've got femininity and a powerful presence, so use them to your advantage. When it comes to things not fitting, yeah, that's no fun. But whatever you do, don't get discouraged. Don't be embarrassed to go up a size or two if you have to—you can always have clothes tailored to fit you perfectly."

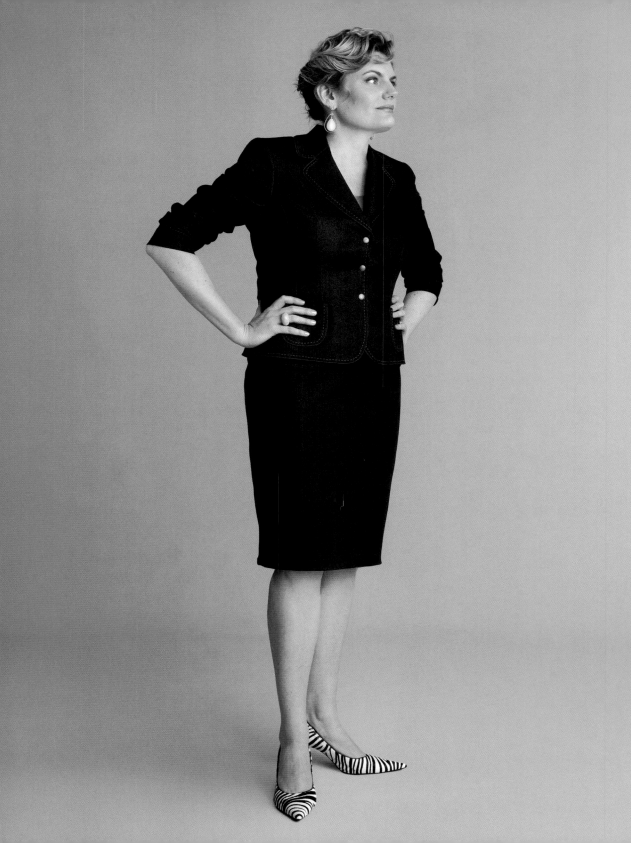

Bigger on Top,
Tall
Work

Wow. Talk about a tall drink of water. See, sometimes keeping things simple can create huge impact. When you've got great height, it's about finding a suit with hourglass structure and letting the tailoring speak for itself.

Look for luxury-fabric suits with a stretch blend. Not only will you feel powerful, but comfortable too.

The three buttons on the jacket help to lock and load The Girls into place, while the pockets on the hip add a little emphasis there, helping you to look less short-waisted.

Here, a straight skirt accentuates the natural curve of the hip and thigh. By keeping the skirt below the knee, we really utilize the natural length of the leg. See the proportion here? It really is like Barbie's: short torso, large chest, and legs a mile long.

When you've got a naturally regal presence, you've got to accessorize with regal jewelry—especially for work and evening. Keep your pieces big and bright to match your stature.

Do not be afraid of a small, we repeat, small shoulder pad in a jacket to help balance a larger chest. This is a particularly effective strategy when you don't have broad shoulders.

Hosiery Option: With super-long legs, you can go with a darker opaque tight, which still keeps a long lean silhouette and balances a larger chest.

Classic or Awful?

Animal prints can be tricky. They can either make you look as sleek as a leopard or as mangy as a junkyard dog. Hopefully these lists will help you figure it out.

ETERNALLY CLASSIC ANIMAL-PRINT PIECES:
- Shoes
- Bag
- Pencil skirt
- Lingerie
- Fabulous vintage ¾-length coat

ETERNALLY AWFUL ANIMAL-PRINT PIECES:
- Leather motorcycle jacket
- Denim jeans
- Linen duster
- Fuzzy slippers

We love a structured ballet slipper (structure meaning "stiffer soled") in a metallic or an interesting color. It's a great weekend shoe with a skirt, jeans, or trousers. And in case you haven't heard the news, metallic for day is just fine.

Shall I compare thee to a summer's day?

Bigger on Top,
Tall
Weekend

A shorter boxy denim jacket in a darker wash helps to downplay the chest considerably.

A scoop-neck knit top opens up the neck area, so you feel feminine without showing cleavage. Plus, knits are a larger-chested woman's best friend; they stretch without buttons pulling.

A cotton A-line skirt in a light color pulls focus to the bottom half of the body, bringing balance to the entire frame.

When it comes to prints, you have got to match the impact of the design to the size of the frame or your look just looks "off." Because Meredith is 5-foot-11, when she chooses to do a floral, she needs to keep it big. If she were 5 feet tall and 98 pounds, she would be completely overwhelmed by this much print. In fact, she'd look like she was being attacked by roses from outer space. And if the print were smaller, she'd look like she was trying too hard to be "dainty."

Universal Tip: Three-quarter sleeves can make taller women look as if they've outgrown their clothes. Try rolling shorter-length sleeves to the elbow for a more purposeful look and a better proportion.

Seasonal Alternative: For colder months, you can easily switch this denim jacket for a wool melton one. Stay away from double-breasted jackets and puffy parkas as they will just make you look top heavier. The cotton skirt could be switched out for a stiffer velvet one. Add patterned tights and knee-high boots, and the outfit takes you into winter.

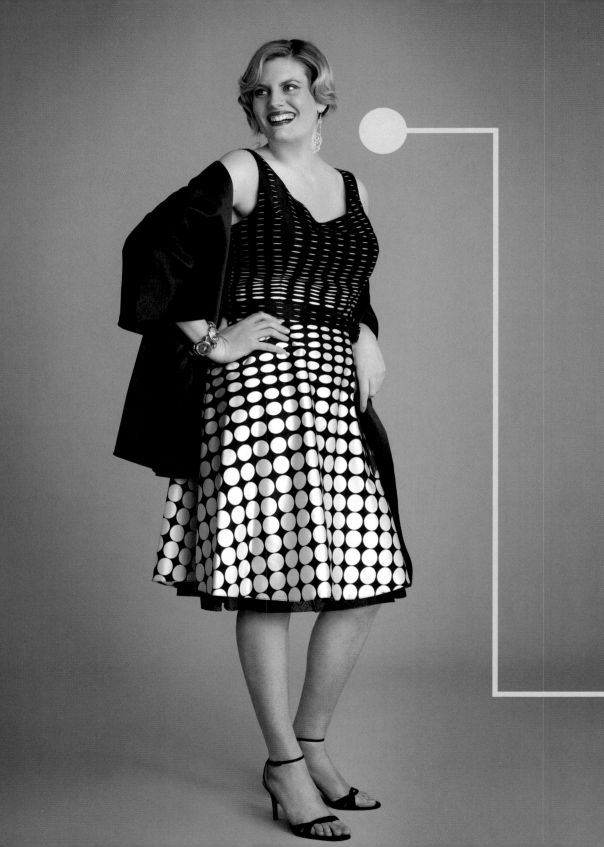

Bigger on Top,
Tall
Evening

First and foremost, a tank **dress** with an A-line skirt is a universally flattering silhouette, regardless of body type. It is particularly flattering for a bustier body type, as it allows for a thicker-strap supportive bra. Anyone who tells you a women with a larger chest should dare to go strapless should be locked up.

The graduating size of the print creates an optical illusion. The bust appears smaller where the print is smaller. As the print gets larger, the eye is drawn downward, balancing the overall body shape.

The sash accents a natural narrowing at the waist and helps to enhance that fab hourglass figure we're always pushing on everyone.

The ankle strap on this high-heel sandal would interrupt the leg line too much on a more petite woman, but on a tall woman it helps to balance the volume of the skirt and just looks downright glamorous in keeping with the entire look.

Universal Tip: Love the dress but feel self-conscious about showing your upper arms? Try a wrap. Some now come with sleeves, but make sure the wrap doesn't compete with the pattern of the dress.

Universal Tip: When wearing black and white for evening, try clear jewelry: rhinestones, crystals, or our favorite, diamonds! Clear stones are eternally chic and don't compete with the bold contrast of black and white.

Foxy!

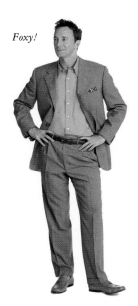

Bigger on the Bottom, Overall

DON'T wear tops that are too long and cover your tush. You only shorten your legs.

DO look for tops that have structure, give you a waistline, and sit above the hip.

MUST-HAVE: A midwidth nonpleated trouser that sits at the top of the hip.

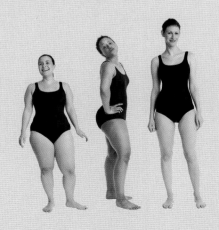

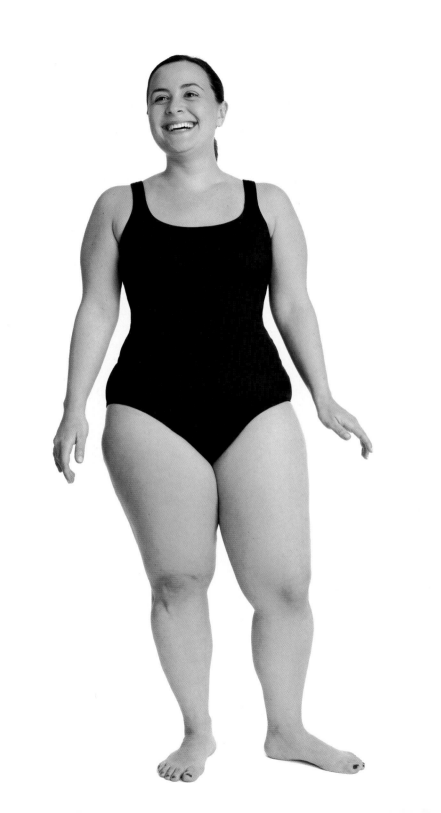

Bigger on the Bottom, Petite

MARNIE
4-foot-11
Size 8 on top
Size 12 on bottom

"My biggest difficulty is in finding pants, particularly jeans, that fit me well. Aside from being petite, I have a much smaller top half and larger bottom half, making it difficult to find pieces that fit correctly everywhere."

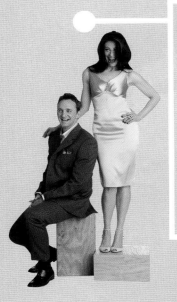

STACY AND CLINTON SAY: "All petites have it rough. They either look childish or grandmotherish (not in the cool, modern grandma kind of way). There just isn't enough out there for them! (Manufacturers, are ya listening?) Add to that, disproportion in a body type, and finding clothes ain't easy. It took even us a while to figure out the best way to dress Marnie's frame! But the result made all of us smile and we all learned something. Keep fluffy details to a minimum. Keep lines clean and architectural. Use flare and seaming on top to balance the bottom, and dance like there's no tomorrow! (See page 46 for Clinton's best moves.)"

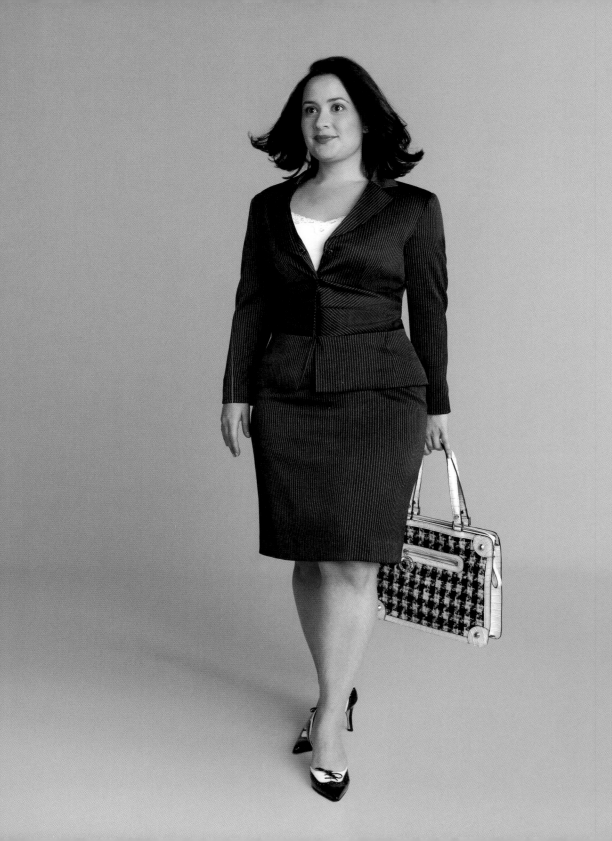

Bigger on
the Bottom,
Petite
Work

We love pinstripes for their subtly elongating effect on the body. When you are petite, this is a great print, which forces the eye to look vertically (creating height) without overwhelming the wearer.

When choosing jackets for this body type it is essential to balance the entire body line. In order to achieve this effect, a small (and we mean small) shoulder pad can help do that. Otherwise, look for a well-seamed and structured shoulder and a high-cut armhole that emphasizes the shoulder without adding bulk.

Look for a jacket with a midlevel stance with a wider lapel and neckline and add a white or light color camisole underneath to keep the attention on the face and chest.

Note the waist seaming on the jacket. It sits slightly higher than the natural waistline, which gives the impression of a longer leg. The seaming is angled, which also creates the impression of a narrower waistline.

The fitted skirt is straight from the widest part of the hip downward. To do an A-line shape here would create added and unnecessary bulk. Marnie's hips are balanced by the peplum (an extension that comes below the waistline) of the jacket. Thus, we get the sleekest, straightest line on the body. The skirt length here goes to the top of the knee, which perfectly balances Marnie's top and bottom halves. To go longer, we would lose the line of her fabulous legs!

Again, being petite, people can assume you are younger. It is important to balance well-fitting clothes with bold and sophisticated accessories. Rely on classics like a houndstooth-print bag or a spectator high **heel** to lend an air of sophistication to any outfit.

Universal Tip: While pointy-toe shoes help to create an even longer leg line (Whew! Look at those gams!), don't feel they have to be boring. A spectator high heel in contrasting colors or a printed shoe will keep the look fresh and current.

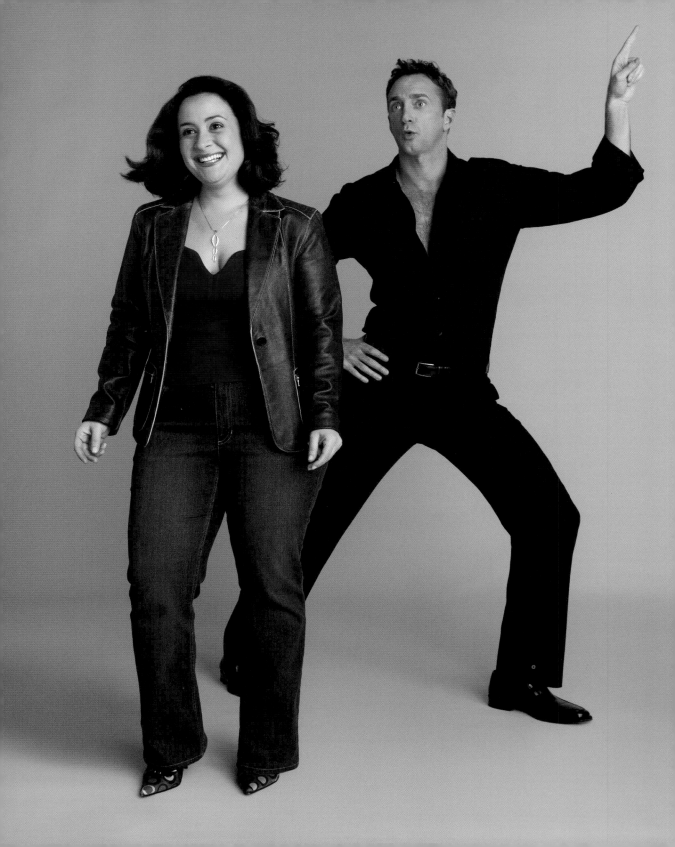

Bigger on the Bottom,
Petite
Weekend

When you are petite and bigger on the bottom, well-fitting jeans can be a tough item to find. Look for a midrise jean to help lengthen the line of the **leg**. Anything too low cut will just make your legs look shorter. Find a jean with a uniform dark wash, which will deemphasize a larger hip or thigh. Avoid at all costs any kind of whiskering or bleaching on or near the hip/thigh region. This just serves to highlight the area we want to play down.

Consider a stretch jean here as long as the leg is straight. The straight cut will help to give you a long leg line but the stretch will slim the leg slightly as well, creating an even lither silhouette. Beware the boot-cut jean. Contrary to what you may have heard, they will only serve to shorten the leg and emphasize the thigh.

Add a heavier weight or stiffer, structured fabric jacket like leather to balance both halves of the body. Make sure the jacket fits well, is snug in the shoulder, and covers the top of the hip for the most flattering effect.

Add a knit sweater in a great color with an interesting neckline and a drop necklace to frame the face and décolleté.

Universal Tip: Don't worry about the length of the jean. If they fit well, ask a tailor to rehem them with the original stitching (no one besides you and your tailor will ever know the difference).

Seasonal Alternative: In winter, a leather jacket won't be enough to keep you warm, but when you are petite and curvy on the bottom, coat proportion is extremely important. If you're like Marnie, look for coats no longer than to the knee and that flare out from the waist slightly. Avoid flap pockets that sit directly on the hip; they just call unwanted attention to the area. But angled slit pockets are quite flattering. Even a '50s looking swing coat is great in terms of length and proportion.

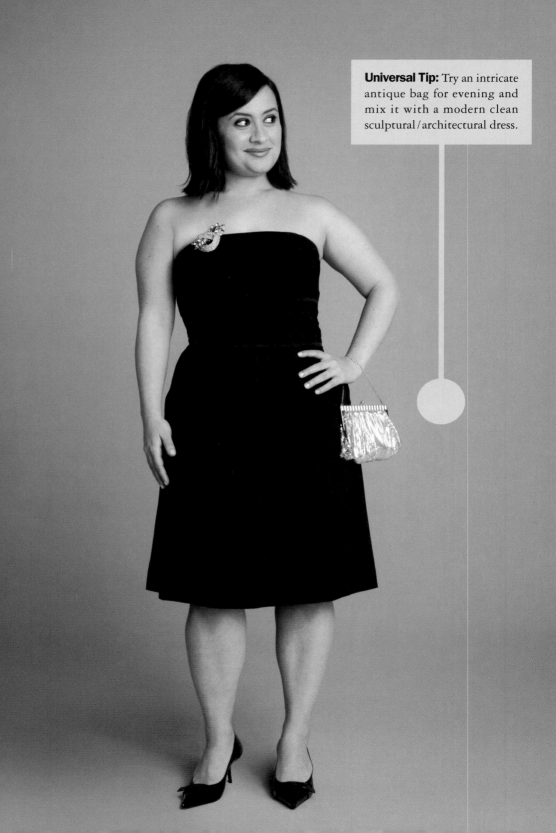

Universal Tip: Try an intricate antique bag for evening and mix it with a modern clean sculptural/architectural dress.

Bigger on the Bottom, Petite
Evening

A strapless dress is a great option for keeping the focus on the shoulders and the upper half of the body. Add a rhinestone brooch for even more dramatic emphasis.

The horizontal seaming at the bust and waist accentuate these areas while the vertical seaming on the skirt serves to lengthen and slim the hip and thigh.

The shape of this dress is a slight but structured A-line. It is almost straight until the midthigh and then slightly bells, making it possible to deemphasize the top of the thigh without losing the line of the body or exaggerating it.

The pointy-toe shoe does not interrupt the line of the leg and the **kitten** heel does not distort her body proportion.

Hosiery Option: When you're as petite as Marnie, you want to show off as much leg as possible. But when you're bigger in the hip and thigh area, a control-top stocking can be a girl's best friend. For evening, stick with sheer or sheer with a seam; anything dark would just weigh down the leg and give Marnie the appearance of being shorter—the last thing we want! (P.S. Always find the closest match between your skin tone and the color of your stockings for the sleekest, most natural appearance.)

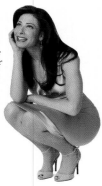

Doesn't Marnie remind you a little of Audrey Hepburn?

Universal Tip: You don't have to wear massively high heels if you are petite. Better to go with a lower heel that is in keeping with the size of your body. Otherwise, you may look like you are walking on stilts (which is a *great* look if you work for the circus).

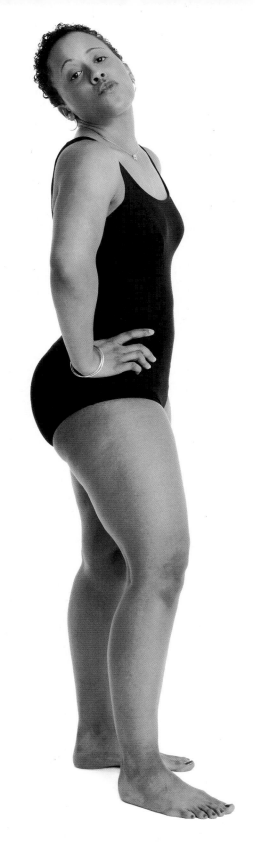

Bigger on the Bottom, Average Height

KIMBERLY

5-foot-4
Size 8 on top
Size 12/14 on bottom

"I've been blessed with junk in my trunk, which I love. But unfortunately, my larger derrière makes it difficult for me to find bottoms that fit well in the waist and hip. Finding dresses is also an issue because my bust is so much smaller in comparison to my lower half."

STACY AND CLINTON SAY: "Curves are great but balance is the key. (Isn't it always?) Because so much of Kim is well proportioned, we can balance the derrière by adding soft layers and volume to other parts of the body without bulking her up. Her body type requires a wider leg, higher-waisted pant, and dresses that have adjustable tops for a proper fit. We also wanted to make sure we focused attention on that face! That smile!"

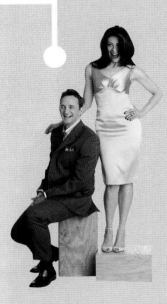

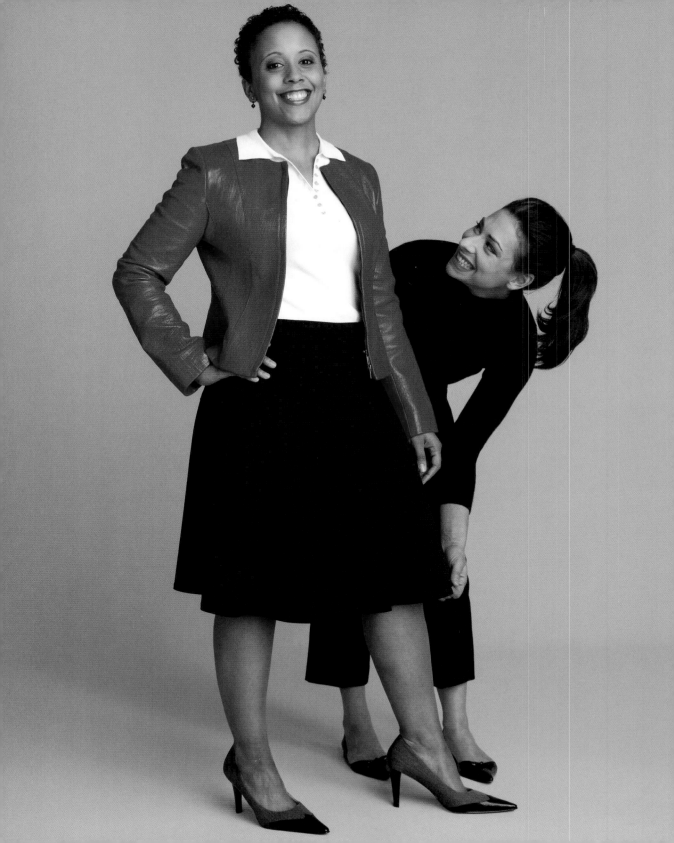

Bigger on the Bottom,
Average Height
Work

Look for A-line skirts that fall away from the body softly in midweight, drapy fabrics in darker colors or subtle prints to deemphasize the hip and derrière.

Use more-impactful colors on the top half (and darker, more neutral colors on the bottom half) to keep the visual focus up on the face and torso while balancing the body shape overall.

Look for a short leather jacket with a strong shoulder line that nips in the waist and sits at the top of the hip to create a longer leg line and slim the hip.

By using two strongly contrasting **colors** (like white on top and black on the bottom), you can create a distinct waistline, and that serves to emphasize an already-narrow waist.

Prominent collars—either on a jacket or a shirt—balance the hip and bookend an outfit.

Hosiery Option: A good choice for Kimberly would be a mid-gray textured hose. Being bigger on the bottom, she won't want to lose the length of her leg, so there should be a bit of (not massive) contrast between her leg and the color of the skirt. And, no, white tights would not balance this outfit. Just banish that thought from your head.

Universal Tip: Pairing red and black can look matronly (very Raiza Gorbachev) but can look infinitely chic with a third color—a neutral such as a white, cream, or camel.

Seasonal Alternative: We loved Kimberly in this red leather jacket, but any fabric with a stiffer construction could work here: tweed, velvet, denim, even cotton canvas for the warmer months. The length and shape of this jacket are what work here, and you could easily pair it with a mid-width trouser or jean if you prefer.

Hardware

While we have no issue mixing metallics in general, it's generally a good idea to stay with the same color on prominent "hardware" in accessories. Here, the belt buckle and metal on the bag are both gold to help the outfit look just a bit more polished.

Bigger on
the Bottom,
Average Height
Weekend

A three-quarter, single-breasted topper coat with subtle waist seaming and a strong shoulder creates a long, straight line by camouflaging the hip area.

Add a **bright**-colored shirt with an exposed neckline or V-neck sweater to add visual interest around the face.

A higher-waisted, slightly wide straight-leg trouser with a belt creates a shorter torso and a longer leg line—which makes everyone look longer and taller!

Believe it or not, women who carry their weight on the lower half find their legs appear shorter. Regardless of height, try on a petite-size pant and you may find it fits you better in the rise.

Always go for a pointy-toed shoe when you're bigger on the bottom. Those with this body type often appear to have longer torsos and shorter legs (the opposite of Barbie!). Wearing a pointy toe keeps the leg looking long and might just inspire you to add "Malibu" in front of your first name.

Universal Tip: Try using "softer" neutrals with brights, instead of black (which has a tendency to look harsh for day), for a more sophisticated color palette. Try chocolate brown, navy, or charcoal gray. They're all still dark and they're just as "slimming" as black.

A note on our choice of bag: The purple bag matches the shirt, which helps make this outfit look cohesive, but a purple bag would be great even if we used a printed shirt with just a bit of purple in it. However, a bold bag that doesn't really match an outfit can still work. Sometimes one contrasting brightly colored accessory can create a whole new look to an outfit. So, be bold!

A general guideline on color and skin tone: Darker and olive skin tones are most flattered by colors with citrus undertones.

Bigger on the Bottom,
Average Height
Evening

When Kimberly put on this dress, even we were astounded. She looked so beautiful in this color! And the cut suits her shape so perfectly. The V-neck halter not only shows off and accentuates beautiful, broad shoulders (and makes the face the focus of the whole outfit), but also can be made smaller by tightening the neck strap.

Because the distinct waistband is made of silk charmeuse (shiny!), it calls attention to itself, emphasizing the narrowness of the waist. Plus, there's a blousing effect created, which balances the width of the hip and thigh.

Again, a softer A-line works here to balance the hip without adding too much volume. The length of the dress balances Kimberly's height while still showing off lots of toned leg.

Hosiery Option: With a dress like this, skin is the *key* element, so sheer hose is really the best option. Or try sheer with a slightly metallic sheen to play up the jewelry choice.

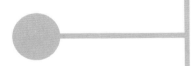

Universal Tip: When choosing accessories for a halter top, pay attention to the thickness of the neck strap. The thicker the strap, the less you need near it. So rather than a necklace, try a great pair of earrings instead.

Ha-cha!

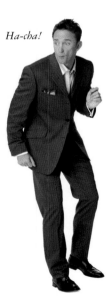

Universal Tip: Metallic shoes are a must-have in every closet for evening—but don't be afraid to wear them during the day!

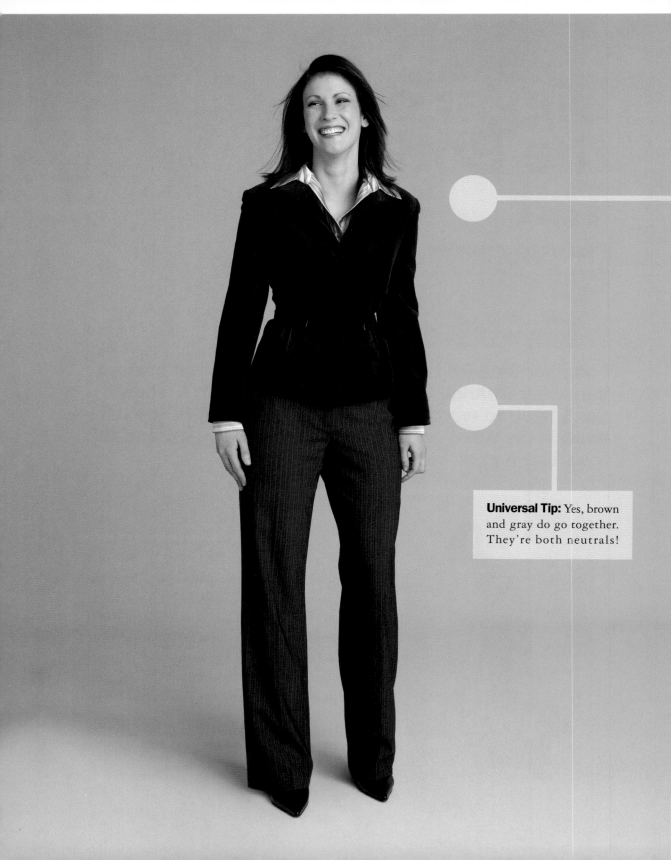

Universal Tip: Yes, brown
and gray do go together.
They're both neutrals!

Bigger on the Bottom,
Average Height
Evening

When Kimberly put on this dress, even we were astounded. She looked so beautiful in this color! And the cut suits her shape so perfectly. The V-neck halter not only shows off and accentuates beautiful, broad shoulders (and makes the face the focus of the whole outfit), but also can be made smaller by tightening the neck strap.

Because the distinct waistband is made of silk charmeuse (shiny!), it calls attention to itself, emphasizing the narrowness of the waist. Plus, there's a blousing effect created, which balances the width of the hip and thigh.

Again, a softer A-line works here to balance the hip without adding too much volume. The length of the dress balances Kimberly's height while still showing off lots of toned leg.

Hosiery Option: With a dress like this, skin is the *key* element, so sheer hose is really the best option. Or try sheer with a slightly metallic sheen to play up the jewelry choice.

Universal Tip: When choosing accessories for a halter top, pay attention to the thickness of the neck strap. The thicker the strap, the less you need near it. So rather than a necklace, try a great pair of earrings instead.

Ha-cha!

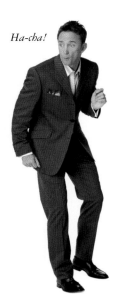

Universal Tip: Metallic shoes are a must-have in every closet for evening—but don't be afraid to wear them during the day!

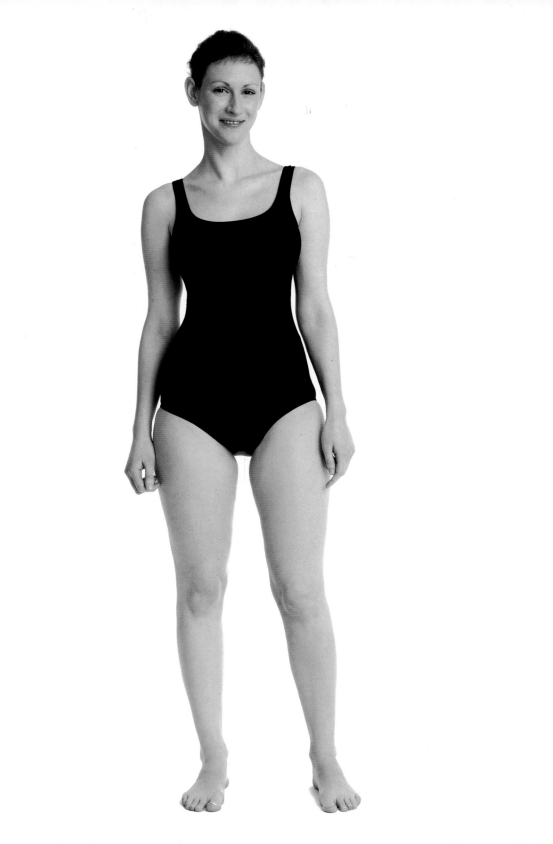

Bigger on the Bottom,
Tall

LEAH
5-foot-9
Size 4 on top
Size 8 on bottom

"I compensate for the difference in my top and bottom halves by wearing low-slung pants and skirts. Then I don't have to worry about finding pieces to fit the difference in my waist and hip. I like my small waist and this feels like a good way to show it off."

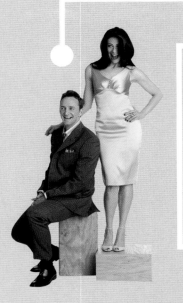

STACY AND CLINTON SAY: "No way! If you carry your weight on the bottom half, chances are your legs look shorter. Wearing low-cut jeans and skirts is just making the issue more noticeable, not less! That lengthens an already-long torso, the opposite of what we want to do. Leah is lucky in that her limbs are long and lean. By emphasizing her arms and legs and creating a higher visual waistline, we can get her looking more proportioned in no time!"

Universal Tip: Yes, brown and gray do go together. They're both neutrals!

Bigger on the Bottom, Tall

Work

Wearing a midrise, midwidth, midweight (*mid* is a big thing with us) **trouser** (this one is a tropical wool with a double pinstripe) deemphasizes the hip because it falls from the widest part of the hip straight down.

The corduroy blazer has a strong shoulder to balance the hip and is elasticized at the waist, creating a cinched (therefore, noticeable) waistline. (A belt worn outside the jacket would be a nice alternative here.) Creating this waistline helps produce that ultra-long-legged Barbie silhouette we love so much.

Get a brightly colored vertical-striped shirt with the collar out to balance the hip and draw attention toward the face.

Don't forget: If your weight is carried in your lower half, pointy-toe shoes always lengthen the leg.

Universal Tip: All right, ladies, we need to talk about the *rise* of your pants. That's right. Right there at the crotch. Please, do not let the crotch of your pant sag down to the middle of your thigh or, God forbid, your knee. For a pant to fit correctly, the rise must sit right at . . . your private bits . . . without any pulling or creasing. If you've got pulls or creases, you've got a pant that doesn't fit you correctly.

Anyone feel like a tall drink of water right now?

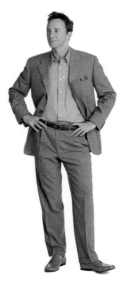

Helpful hint: With heavier hips and legs, a strong shoulder can be reemphasized by altering and narrowing the sleeves of a jacket.

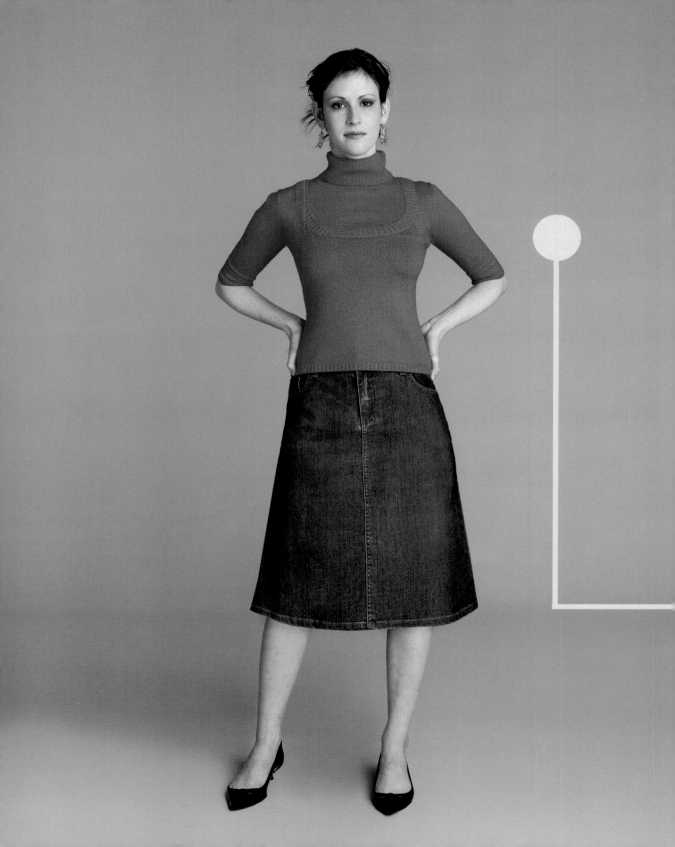

Bigger on the Bottom,
Tall
Weekend

Outfits don't need to be complicated to work. Just look at Leah—two pieces with the right cut and shape for her figure.

Start with a top in a brighter color to add visual interest to the top half and to trick the eye, leading it upward toward the face and shoulder.

Look for a turtleneck, which can deemphasize a long neck and add volume to a small-framed torso.

This sweater is stitched to appear as if it is a double layer without being too bulky. Choose a three-quarter sleeve to focus attention at the waistline. The sleeve ends just at the waist, accentuating it. The sweater hits just at the top of the hip, lessening the difference in proportion between the waist and the hip.

Choose a stiffer denim skirt to create a stronger, straighter A-line silhouette. This kind of fabric camouflages a hip most distinctly. It does the work of creating the shape of the hip rather than relying on the actual shape of the hip.

Because of Leah's height, high heels aren't a necessity. (But we always love tall girls in high heels! We love all girls in heels!) A pointy-toed flat still elongates a heavier leg.

Universal Tip: The illusion of a double-layer knit helps to balance out a wider bottom. Look for layering pieces on top to balance the entire body line.

Seasonal Alternative: You could wear this kind of outfit all year long. For spring, as you see it here. For fall, add tights to wear with the flats and look for coats that fit snugly in the shoulder. A short puffy parka would keep the leg line long—as would a great double-breasted short pea coat.

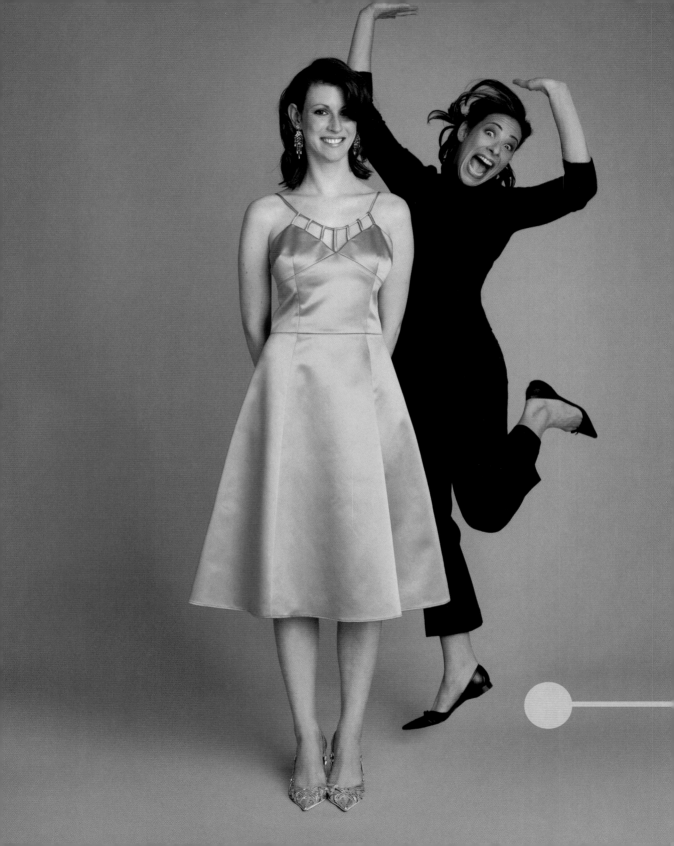

Bigger on the Bottom, Tall
Evening

Dutchess satin has a fairly heavy weight. It is a stiffer fabric, perfect for intricate seaming and construction. It has more structure and much less sheen than charmeuse, making it an ideal fabric for camouflaging areas of the body. It also takes **color** very well, resulting in a range of beautiful hues.

Look for this kind of detailing at the neckline: it helps to broaden the shoulder for overall body balance and accents the face, neck, and décolleté.

The angled seaming beneath the breast accents a narrow torso and the horizontal waist seam helps to raise the visual center of gravity, resulting in our favorite combo (drum roll, please): a shorter torso and a longer leg line!

Strong vertical seaming on the skirt emphasizes height, and the actual volume on this skirt deemphasizes the hip area completely.

Because we've created a longer leg line with a high waist seam, high heels aren't essential here. We've paired this dress with a silver kitten-heel sling-back that doesn't interrupt the line of the leg.

Universal Tip: A beautiful color is a wonderful option for cocktail hour rather than the ubiquitous black. If you've got pale skin, go with lighter colors; darker skin, go brighter.

Universal Tip: When your dress is all about architecture (i.e., clean lines), it's nice to juxtapose that with a softer bag. Try something unconstructed or, better yet, a poufy feather ball-shaped bag!

A Little Extra in the Middle, Overall

DON'T accentuate your thinner legs with skinny pants and skirts. Your top half will look even larger by comparison.

DO look for tops with structure and bottoms with a little bit of volume to help proportion a midsection.

MUST-HAVE: A one- or two-button fitted jacket with a stance that hits above the natural waistline.

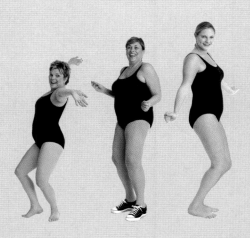

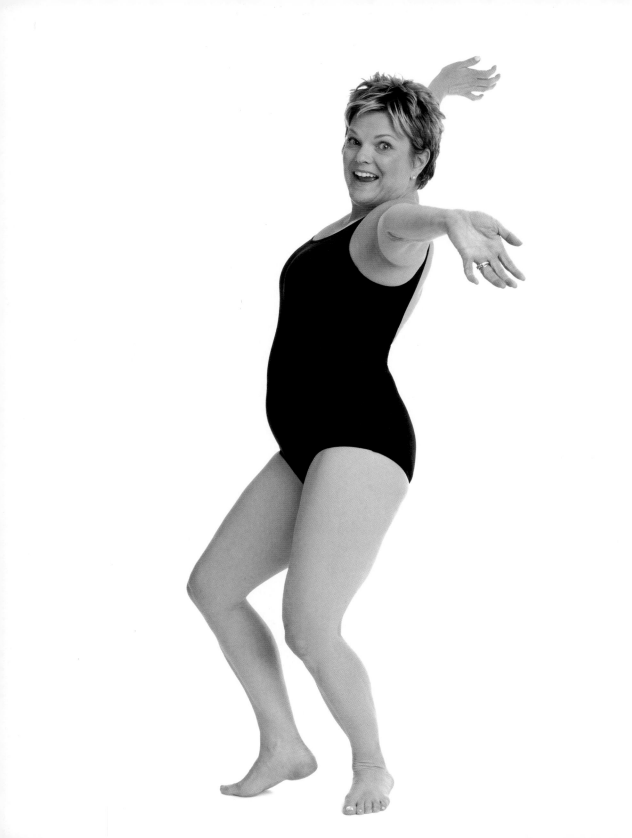

A Little Extra in the Middle, Petite

KRISTINA
5-foot-3
Size 8/10

"I have two major frustrations. The first is finding blouses that actually button without pulling everywhere. Anything that fits my back and shoulders makes me look frumpy because the cut is so large! But anything that clings gives me more of a tummy. And second, everything is too long. I am forever altering everything. I do have one long-sleeve T-shirt, which is my favorite item of clothing. It fits my back and shoulders and trims my waistline to show I have curves and am not built like an igloo."

STACY AND CLINTON SAY: "Alteration is not your enemy. Until manufacturers make more variety in petite sizes, you are stuck. Accept this and move on! When you have a broad back and a tummy, it is important to find clothes that deemphasize that width and create a more hourglass silhouette. One word: jackets. And when you're petite, that's really three words: structured, short jackets. They will make up for any body line imbalance. Also, use a broad back and shoulders to your advantage. Rather than fighting them, show them off to balance your midsection."

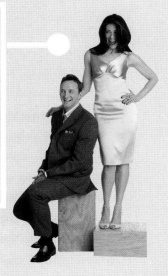

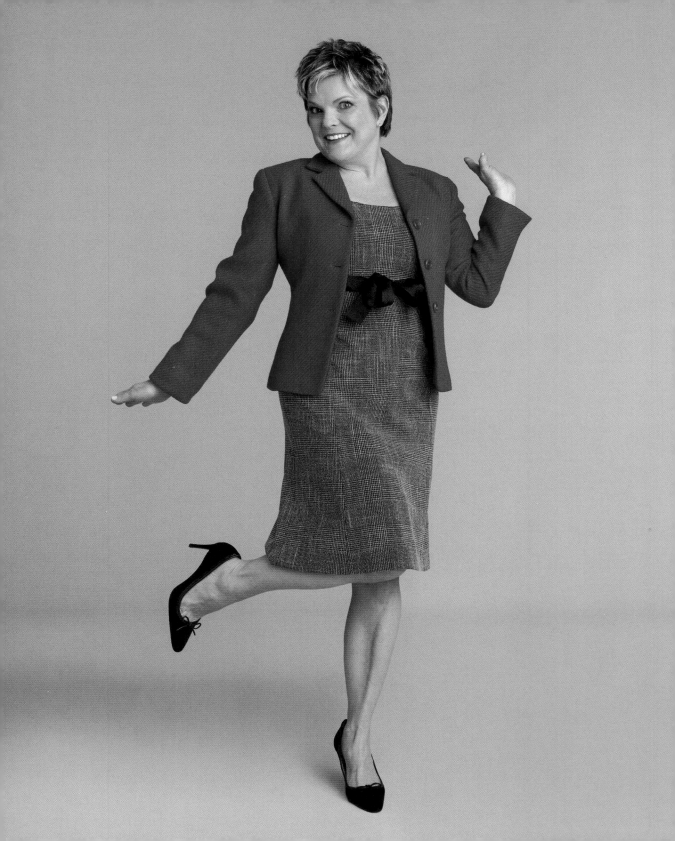

A Little Extra
in the Middle,
Petite

Work

Start with a jacket in a beautiful color, then take a look at the shape: does it curve in at the waistline or is it boxy?

Look for a jacket that gives the shape of two mirror-image Cs on your torso. It nips in at the waist, creating a smaller waistline, and falls over the top of the hip to add extra emphasis to the curve while also adding separation between the arm and the torso.

Look for jackets with a high-set armhole so that it fits closely to the shoulder, which deemphasizes a broader frame.

Dresses with an empire waist deflect the eye upward toward the chest and away from the natural waist. The emphasis is on the top of the rib cage, which is the narrowest part of the torso.

Raising the eye line to a higher part of the torso gives the illusion of a longer line on the body, which is particularly helpful if you're petite.

Try a fitted, yet slightly A-line **dress** to balance the width of the midsection. (If the cut were narrower, the tummy would become the focus and look like the widest part of the body.)

A midheight skinny heel with a pointy toe elongates the leg line, helping to balance a wider shoulder and midsection.

Universal Tip: Suits don't have to be a jacket-and-pant or jacket-and-skirt combo. Look for a jacket-and-dress combination. It's a very feminine look and sometimes more flattering than the former two.

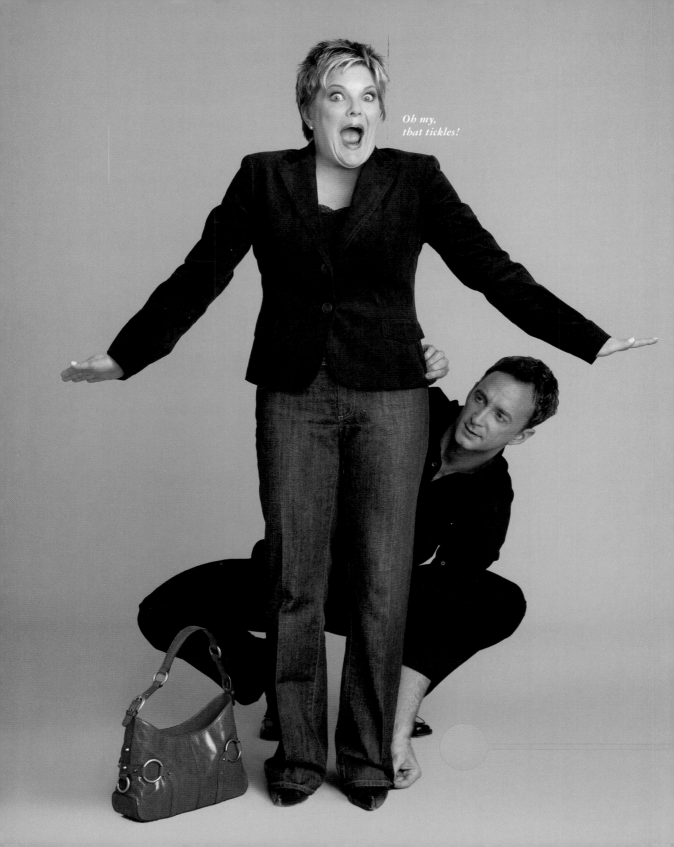

Oh my,
that tickles!

A Little Extra in the Middle,
Petite
Weekend

This structured short blazer has a two-button closure with a midlevel stance that hits between the tummy and the breast line.

The chocolate brown color is in contrast to Kristina's eyes and complexion and make them pop.

The midsection is slimmed by the cinch of the bottom button without pulling!

Look for jackets that sit no lower than the top of the hips.

A slight shoulder pad can work here to balance out a thicker middle. When you are petite, creating a bit more length in the overall body is ideal. Add a shoulder pad only to lengthen the distance between the shoulder and a thicker midsection.

Make sure the jacket has a narrow sleeve (even if that means altering it to make it slimmer) to keep the appearance of volume on the top half to a minimum and the limbs looking lean.

Stick to a uniform wash on a midwidth, midrise denim trouser for the longest leg length. A denim trouser can look more sophisticated and age-appropriate than a "regular" jean.

Add a pointy-toe boot to heighten this effect.

Petites should beware the superpointy toe, however. Without some height to carry it off, it can look disproportionate to the rest of you.

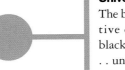

Universal Tip: The jacket is brown. The bag is orange. This is an attractive color combo as opposed to black and orange. Too Halloween . . . unless it is Halloween. Then by all means, knock yourself out.

Universal Tip: The width of the pant matches and balances the width of the shoulder and midsection. We're not big fans of the traditional five-pocket straight jean with creases on the leg. (It's kinda nerdy, to be honest.) But we're all for creases on a trouser leg (denim or otherwise) to keep legs looking their lankiest.

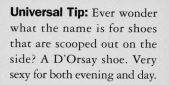

Universal Tip: Ever wonder what the name is for shoes that are scooped out on the side? A D'Orsay shoe. Very sexy for both evening and day.

A Little Extra
in the Middle,
Petite
Evening

Talk about making Kristina's eyes sparkle! The **color** of this dress truly complements her coloring! It echoes, rather than contrasts with, her eyes.

Add turquoise jewelry near the face to really create a striking impact.

If you have strong shoulders, try a spaghetti strap to emphasize them and the décolleté. The rest of the body (especially a midsection) looks much narrower by comparison.

A shorter hemline in front and the longer one in back give extra length to the leg.

Inverted tiers and alternating fabrics create the illusion that you are longer and narrower . . . like a tall glass of water.

Look for dresses in alternating fabrics like this—the shiny (silk charmeuse) and matte (chiffon) fabrics create an optical illusion of the tummy being slimmer while the dress has some volume.

The actual line of this dress is straight but the triangular tiers make it appear as if it bells slightly because of their angle. The line of the body looks narrower in comparison. (See Curvy Tall, page 117, for more of this example.)

> **Universal Tip:** Try pairing a brightly colored cocktail dress with a shoe in a similar tonal range but contrasting color. Both Kristina's dress and shoe have the same brightness but are opposite colors. The effect is sophisticated and fresh for evening.

Seasonal Alternative: Two things to think about if you want to wear a dress like this in colder weather:
• Keep the stockings sheer and nude; anything else will distract from the dress and draw the eye downward, making you appear shorter.
• Look for a single-breasted coat that comes to the hem of the dress. The effect will look like one long column, creating a sense of height and a lean body shape.

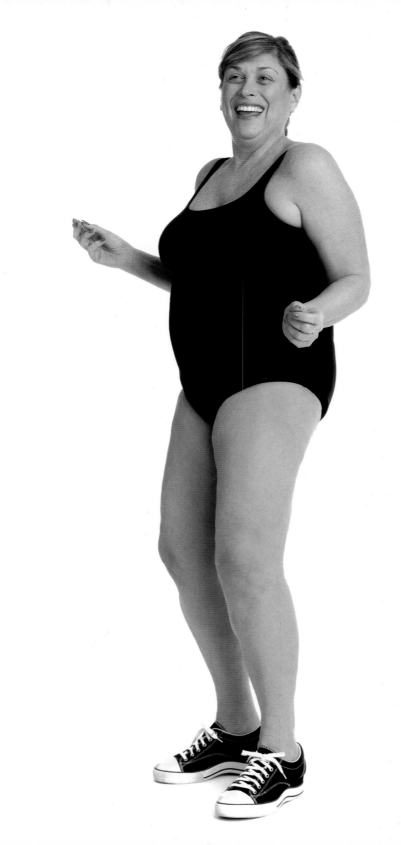

A Little Extra in the Middle,
Average Height

BETTE

5-foot-7

Size 16

"My waist is too large, period. Pants are difficult for me to buy because my waist is a size 16 and my hips are a size 14. I love my low-waisted jeans because they fit me the best. My favorite body part is my butt because from behind I appear smaller than I am."

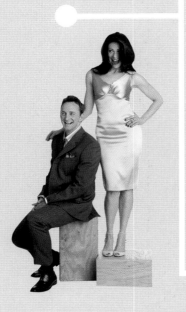

STACY AND CLINTON SAY: "If your favorite body part is your butt just because it appears smaller from behind, then Houston, we have a problem. How is anyone going to see Bette's beautiful face if she's walking around backward all the time? Clearly, if Bette struggles with her midsection, then we have to work to slim it by changing the silhouettes she's been wearing. A low-rise jean is probably not the way to go, because low-rise shortens the leg and makes the midsection look wider. In addition, when your waist size is larger than your hip size, always go with the larger size. You have to fit the biggest part of you first; otherwise nothing can fit properly. Bette has a short torso and long legs, so we want to capitalize on that proportion."

Universal Tip: If there's a slight (and we mean slight) natural pull at the buttons due to breast or tummy size, but you feel the shirt fits well, have Velcro or small hidden snaps sewn in between the buttons so that the shirt lies flat.

Bling Thing

In general, the richness of jewel tones complements mature skin. Brights can play up imperfections as the skin ages and neutrals can not only wash skin out, but they get boring after a while. Choose colors with the names of jewels—sapphire, ruby, emerald, amethyst—and you'll look like you're worth as much as these lovely rocks cost!

A Little Extra in the Middle,
Average Height
Work

First, we had to get Bette a real pair of trousers that sit on her natural waistline!

To balance the midsection, always go with a slightly wider straight leg.

Ideally, look for trousers with a crease for a strong vertical line.

We always say that a structured jacket is basically the solution to everything, but in this case a stretch silk shantung shirt worked just as well! The stiffness of the fabric and the flattering cut of the shirt give the appearance of a more hourglass shape.

The shoulder seam of the shirt should fit squarely at the edge of the shoulder. If the seam falls past the shoulder, the shirt is too big and will just add volume to the top half of the body.

For an overall balanced look in the torso, look for shirts with small side vents, which create a slight flare.

Note the length of the shirt shouldn't go longer than the top of the hip.

With a button-down, open up the neck for a nice V and instantly elongate the neckline and frame the face.

The amethyst color complements Bette's hair and skin color and works well with a softer neutral like gray.

Seasonal Alternative: When you find a pair of trousers in a three-season fabric, which means the only time you probably couldn't wear these would be in the dead of summer, there are lots of alternatives you can pair with them. Think about:
- A schweater that doesn't have prominent ribbing at the waistline for when the weather gets cooler.
- A great V-neck sweater to keep attention up by the face.
- A twin set—knit shell with matching cardigan.

Of course, a fitted blazer in a light tweed will look great over this top.

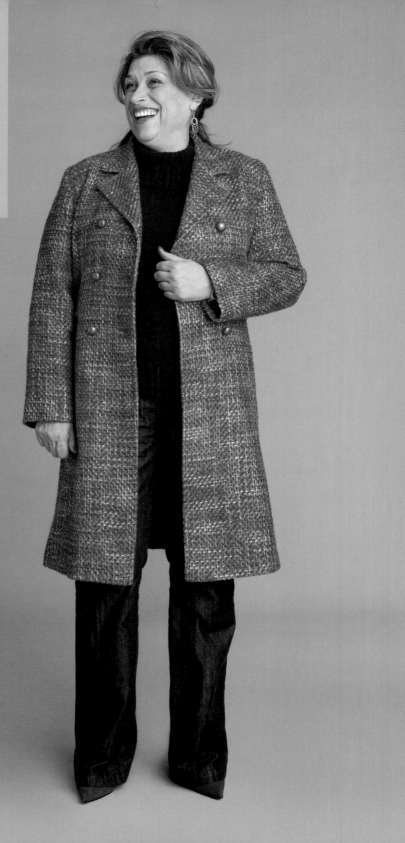

Color Theory

Want to wear different colors together but not sure how? Start with one item that is multicolored, like our tweed coat. Match other items to these colors and round out the outfit with one or two neutrals, like the red boots. We only wish we had a yellow bag to add to the mix!

A Little Extra in the Middle,
Average Height
Weekend

When Bette walked out in this outfit, Clinton exclaimed she looked like Catherine Deneuve. It doesn't get much better than that, does it?

Colored tweed has a real richness to it. It can go from the office to evening, but we love it paired with denim for the weekend. It's so Coco. (Chanel, that is.)

Look for a three-quarter, not full-length, tweed trench when you are average height. Full-length tweed can look bulky and overwhelm your frame.

A coat with a silk or nylon lining will ensure that a wool tweed won't bulk up against your clothing (especially knitwear) and will fall properly against the body.

Try sweaters with a slightly looser weave (which doesn't cling) and avoid tight or thick ribbing at the waistline.

By wearing a darker sweater and dark wide-leg jean, you create a narrow-column silhouette framed by the bright coat.

Wear the coat open to create a long vertical column down the front of your body—very slimming.

The pointy red boot pulls the whole look together!

Thank you, Bette, for wearing boots a little too small for you just 'cause that outfit was fab! The things we do for love . . . of shoes!

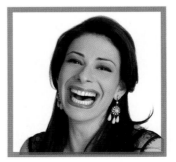

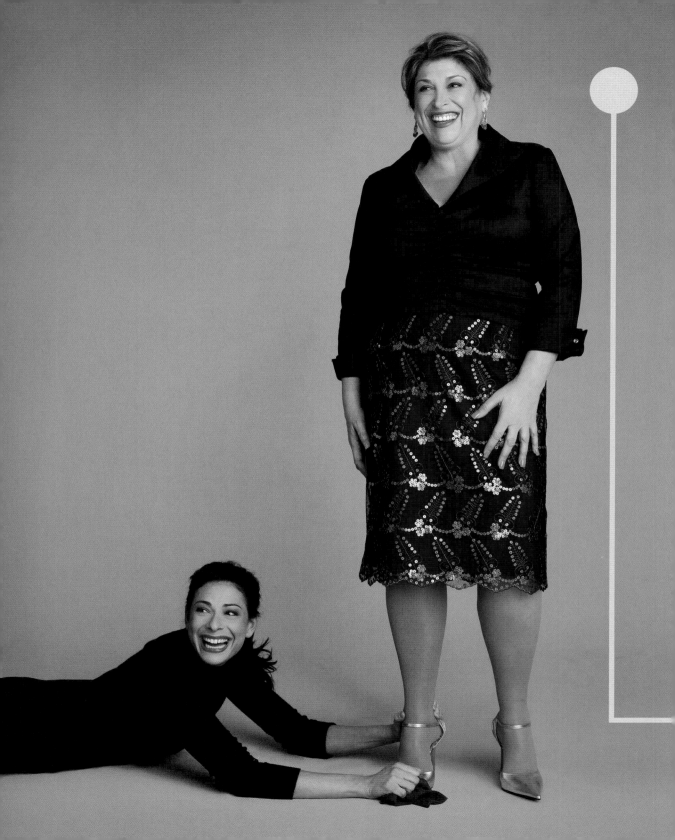

A Little Extra in the Middle,
Average Height
Evening

The key to this outfit is to work with the natural proportion of Bette's body: a short torso and long legs.

Look for a blouse in a stiffer stretch material. This will hold the body shape.

The ruching in a vertical line down the center of the torso acts to cinch in the waist.

The slightly wider cut sleeve keeps the torso balanced with a wider midsection.

Always try a V-neck with a prominent collar to bring attention up toward the face.

By bisecting the body just at the widest part of the midsection (against natural instinct), the tummy can be camouflaged. The length of this skirt highlights a short torso and splits up the midsection. (Head on, just like we said.)

To trick the eye, pair the shirt with a patterned skirt. The focus becomes the lower half of the body.

Use length to balance width. If you carry weight in the top half of your body, you must cover enough of the leg to balance that top half and to look leaner. Otherwise you will have the marshmallow-on-toothpicks look. Not good, trust us.

Bette has long legs and so using an ankle strap doesn't adversely affect the line of the leg, plus a pointy shoe still keeps the line long.

Universal Tip: Go crazy for evening. Mix your metallics! With this burgundy, both silver and gold play equal yet complementary roles.

Universal Tip: When trying to detract from the midsection, think about wearing your hair up for the evening, add some chandelier earrings, and lengthen your neckline!

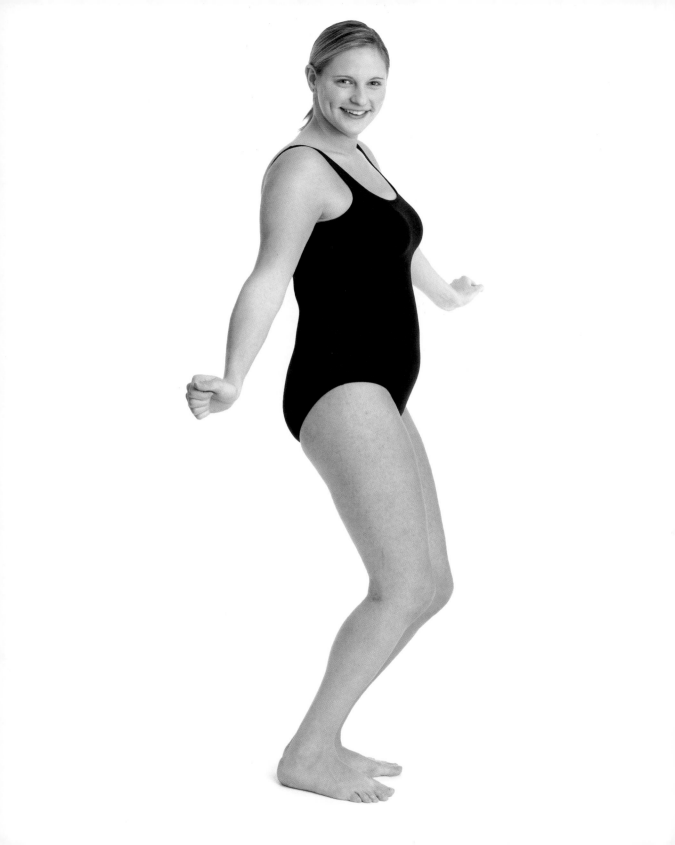

A Little Extra in the Middle,
Tall

JENNIFER
5-foot-11
Size 14

"I think what's most difficult about dressing my body is that cute little roll I get right above the waist of my pants—when I gain a few pounds, it goes straight to my tummy. I get a little self-conscious about it sometimes and try to cover it up with looser sweaters. I love to play up my height and my super-long legs—find me a pair of pants that is actually long enough (it's harder than it sounds) and I will strut my stuff in them all day long."

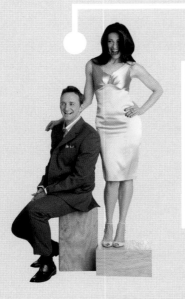

STACY AND CLINTON SAY: "Wow, you're not kidding about the long legs. Jennifer's inseam is 35 inches! When it comes to pants, your first question will probably always have to be: Can they be let out a little? (Or a lot.) As for 'that cute little roll,' we can hide that pretty easily. The trick is not so much looser sweaters as it is longer shirts and structured jackets."

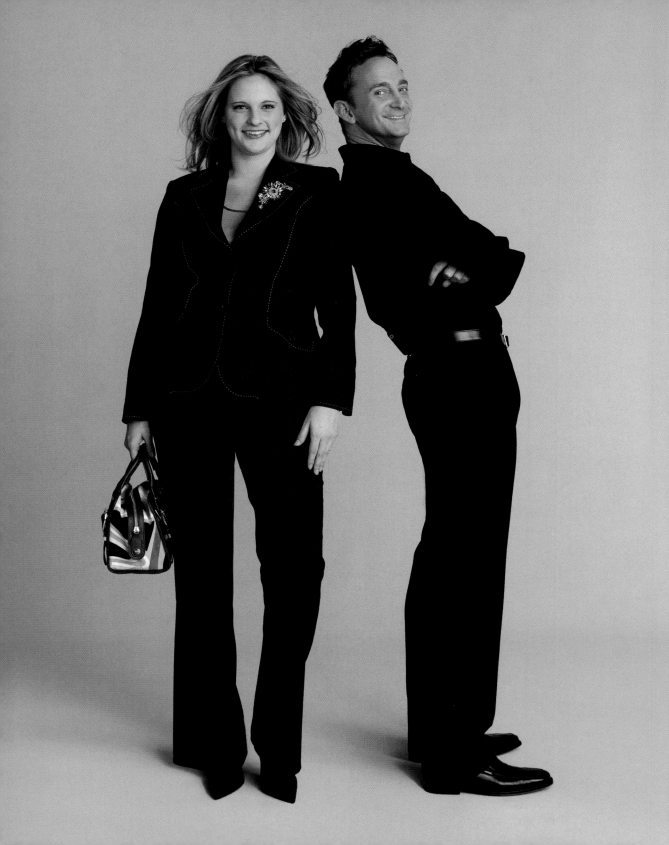

A Little Extra in the Middle,
Tall

Work

This two-button jacket helps pull everything into place. Your jacket shouldn't be tight on the tummy but should create a line that narrows at the waist.

The angled vertical seaming down the length of the torso and angled position of the pockets both contribute to the illusion of an hourglass shape.

The jacket length hits Jennifer right *below* her hip bone, which helps to balance the entire length of her body and streamlines a thicker midsection.

We direct the focus to Jennifer's face by adding a top with a shot of color underneath the suit and a large multicolored **brooch** on the lapel.

The slight flare on the pant doesn't cut the line of the leg when the leg is this long! Add a pointy boot and we still get miles of leg and a stylish silhouette.

We always say match the size of the accessories to the stature of the frame you are dressing. But another option is to go with a bold print—regardless of size—to balance a bigger frame.

Universal Tip: All accessories have the power to dress up an outfit. Jewelry is no exception. Biggest statements? Here are our top five picks:
- Brooches
- Bangle bracelets
- Multiple-chain necklaces
- Cocktail rings
- Chandelier earrings

Universal Tip: Add some fun to a muted-color work suit with bold accessories. And who can resist a Pucci handbag? Not us!

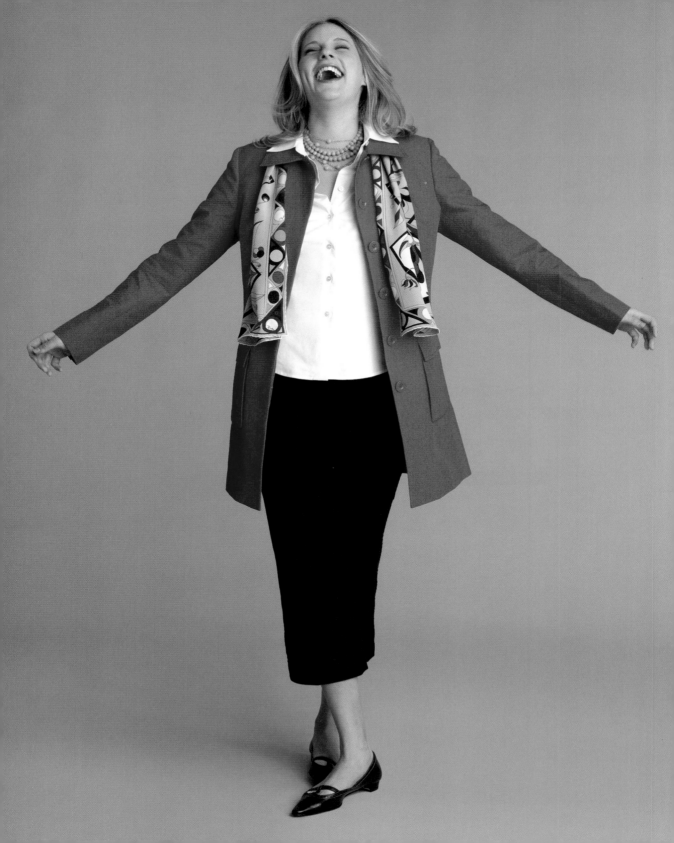

A Little Extra in the Middle,
Tall
Weekend

When you're tall and carry a little extra tummy weight low on the body, go for a button-front shirt that doesn't narrow at the hem, but falls away from the body with a somewhat boxy construction.

Choose a slightly higher-waisted, wider straight pant. The higher waist helps cover a little bit of tummy. (Low rises can create tummies where none exist, so imagine what they do when you have a "cute little roll.") Adding a little width in the pant helps to balance out what's above it.

Jennifer can do a cropped pant with ease because at **5-foot-11** she has plenty of leg to keep her line long.

A brightly colored trench that covers your hip to the top of the thigh keeps a nice straight line and camouflages the midsection of the body. We keep the focus up on the top half with some bright beads, a nice-sized collar on both the shirt and the trench, and a graphic scarf. Again, Pucci seems to be a theme. Hmmm.

Universal Tip: When you're supertall but still want length of line in the leg, go for a pointed ballet flat or Mary Jane.

Seasonal Alternative: Wanna try a cropped pant for fall? Start with a heavier-weight fabric and a knee-high boot. Warning! Your boot *must* clear the hem of the pants. We shouldn't see skin anywhere on the leg.

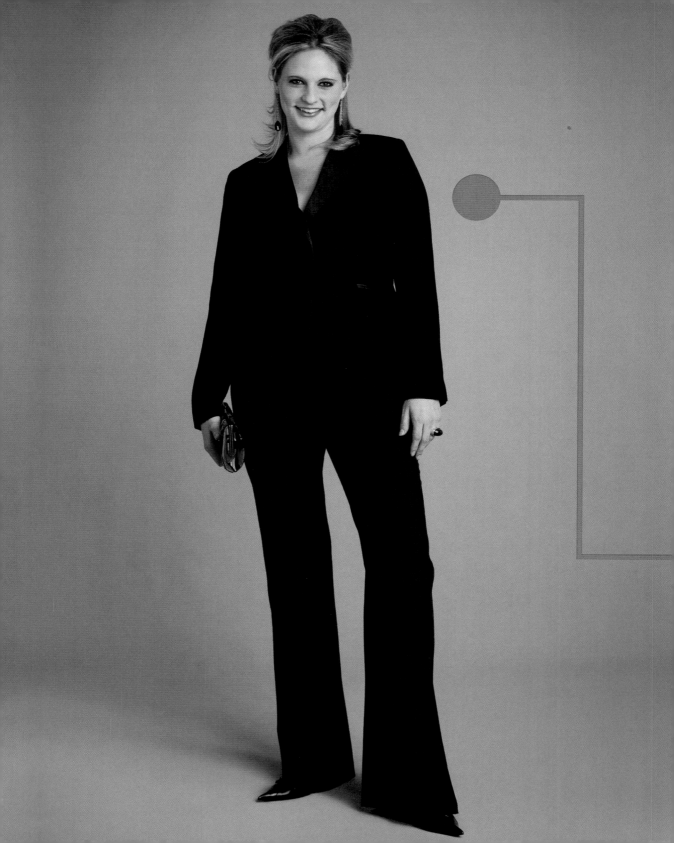

A Little Extra in the Middle,
Tall
Evening

To make the most use of height and camouflage a tummy at the same time, we love a tuxedo for evening. It's a great alternative to a cocktail dress and makes a powerful statement: strong but super sexy at the same time.

When doing one color from head to toe, you can do a slightly shorter jacket. To make sure you still hide the tummy, look for a one-button jacket with a high stance that hits just beneath the breast line, at the narrowest part of the torso. It creates a leaner line and still allows for some room in the midsection.

Look for a tux with a contrasting fabric on the lapel to keep attention up by the face and raise the glamour quotient.

When you've already got long legs, a long boot-cut trouser balances the width of the midsection and yet still allows for that leggy statuesque silhouette.

The large cocktail ring and the drop earrings are both simple, yet their size is in keeping with her stature, and they don't pull focus from this outfit's simple and elegant impact.

Universal Tip: No need for an underpinning for an evening tux. Bare skin is bold and sexy.

Hmm, why didn't I think to wear that?

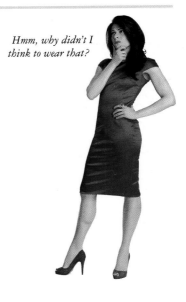

Evening Alternative: Try a white tux. Just make sure it is tailored to perfection. Very Bianca Jagger à la 1970s Studio 54, and guaranteed to turn heads.

Curvy,
Overall

DON'T attempt to wear super-low-rise items. They will accent your hips and give you love handles!

DO look for items that follow your natural curves and accent the narrowness of your waistline.

MUST-HAVE: A wrap or faux wrap dress in cotton or nylon jersey fabric. The wrap dress accents a great waist and natural curves without clinging to them.

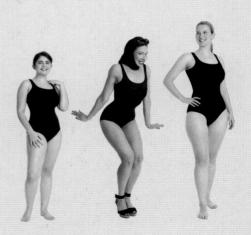

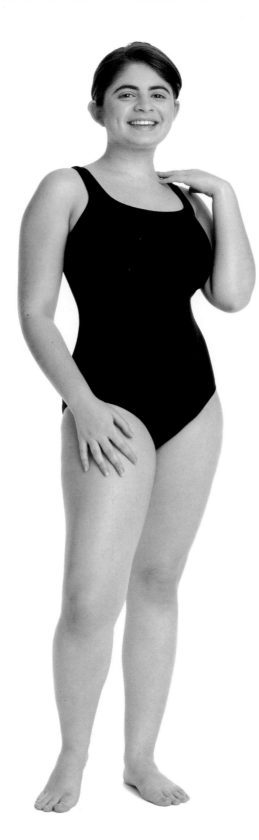

Curvy,
Petite

MARINA
5-foot-2
Size 6

"I have trouble finding clothes that fit all the parts of my body at the same time. Pants that fit me in the hips never fit my waist, and dresses are a particular problem. If they fit me in the chest, they are far too big from the waist down, and a good fit from the waist down is impossible to zip up around the chest! Even if I find a great piece that fits my chest and waist and hips, it is always too long for my body and needs lots of hemming. I would love to wear strappy, more revealing tops but find it difficult with a chest my size. I like having all the curves and I really like my shoulders and upper back, I just wish instead of always covering up I could show them off!"

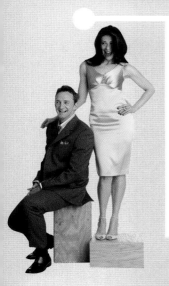

STACY AND CLINTON SAY: "Let's face it. Being petite makes finding clothes you love tricky, but petite with the curves of the average sizes? Now we're talking tough. It can be difficult in the extreme to find pieces that work with your shape and still maintain a lean line. Fortunately, having curves on both the top and bottom gives your body automatic proportion. The key is to keep your limbs looking long, while defining and emphasizing your shoulders and small waist. And hey, petites in particular must use the services of a tailor! Don't miss out on a flattering pair of pants because they are too long. If they fit everywhere else, hemming is the easy part."

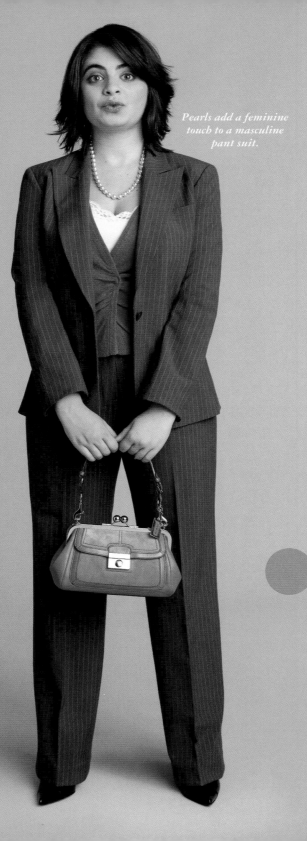

Pearls add a feminine touch to a masculine pant suit.

Curvy,
Petite
Work

Pinstripe is an ideal pattern for petites. It is a vertical stripe, creating a longer body impression. This allows you to give the impression of elongation so that you do not look stout.

Look for a slightly longer lapel on a one-button jacket to give more surface area to the torso and to slightly deemphasize lots of curves without hiding them completely.

Notice this jacket falls to the bottom of the hip, but you can keep the leg long by wearing the jacket open and layering with underpinnings that hit at the waistline.

When layering with thin **knits,** look for one with vertical ruching to call attention to a narrow waist.

A midwidth straight trouser with a crease balances the hip and thigh and elongates the leg—with the help of our trusty pointed shoe!

Universal Tip: Try layering underneath a jacket with a camisole and a thin knit. Layering gives depth to an outfit and helps it to look more polished.

Universal Tip: Remember to look for accessories that are proportionate to your size. Smaller lady, smaller bag.

Seasonal Alternative: As it gets warmer, you may want to peel off the sweater layer seen here. Try a silk camisole in a great color to get the same effect and keep a nice long line at the neck. Also, for a "springier" feel, look for an open-toe sandal with a heel.

Animal print for day?
Sure. Think of animal
print as a neutral.
Matches with brown,
black, tan, and cream,
but also pops against
bright colors.

Curvy,
Petite
Weekend

A slightly shorter, boxier three-button jacket locks and loads The Girls and calls attention to a small waistline.

Make sure the **jacket** molds to the curve of the hip or just sits on top of the hip to keep your body proportionate.

Look for darker sweaters with a contrasting waistband to keep emphasis on a narrow waistline and a long leg line. (We recommend the best cashmere you can afford. It lasts longer and doesn't pill as much or as quickly as wool.) If you are worried that covering your neck makes you look shorter, try a crewneck instead of a turtleneck.

Think about a pair of wider-leg jeans that look more like trousers. Fit them from the widest part of the hip, straight down. They have a defined waistband and have a more polished look that can work in some professional settings as well. They deemphasize curves but still keep legs looking long.

We've shown a pointy shoe, but another alternative for weekend is a soft leather loafer or "driving shoe." While not pointy, these shoes generally have an elongated toe box that balances the leg line as well.

Universal Tip: A tweed jacket is totally multipurpose. Sassy with denim on the weekends and professional with solid skirts or trousers at work!

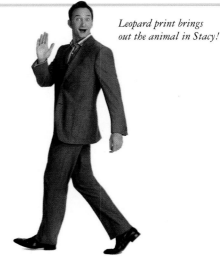

Leopard print brings out the animal in Stacy!

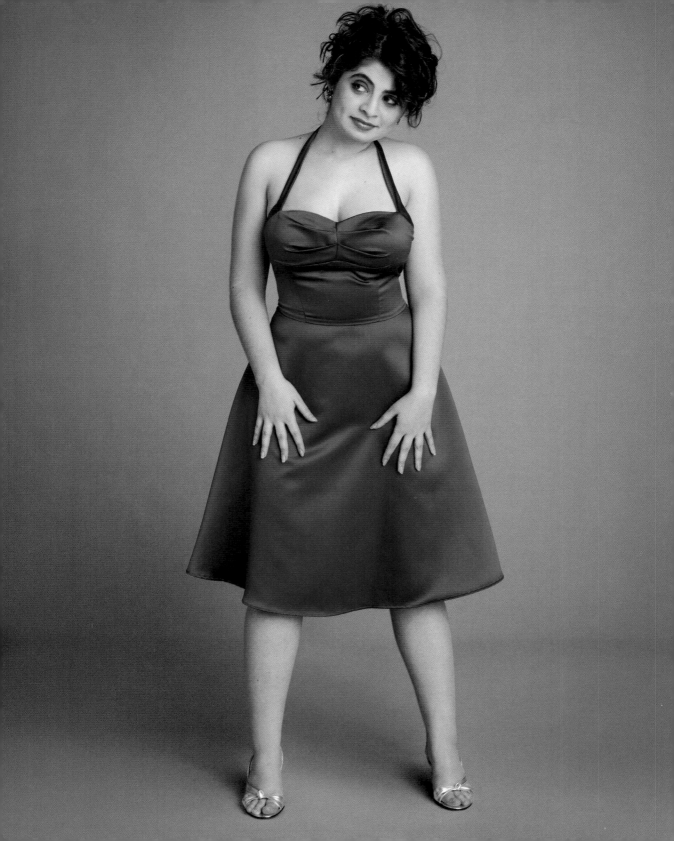

Curvy, Petite
Evening

This is an example of using all your curves to their best advantage. We couldn't get over how stunning Marina looked in this **color** and the dress seemed as if it had been made for her.

Dutchess satin is structured and has enough weight to support curves and show them off.

The halter neck with seamed bustline accentuates the bust but fully supports it as well.

There is an empire seam and a waist seam, which highlight a narrow waist but also create a corset effect to hold the chest in place.

The A-line skirt of the dress does not completely camouflage the hip but slims it within the structured volume of the skirt, hinting at the body line in the most flattering and sexy way.

Play up your hourglass silhouette by wearing clothes made for that body type: the 1950s-style was tailor-made for you. Add vintage jewelry in a matching or boldly contrasting color to complete the feel.

We love metallic shoes with colored satin outfits. The contrast is eye catching, but remember, super-high heels when you are petite is not necessary and can make a curvy body look heavier. Stick to kitten-sized heels, and steer clear of ankle straps. Go for a pump or sling-back. We want that leg to look as long as possible, and the best way to do so is to keep the line uninterrupted.

Universal Tip: For all brunettes with pale skin: Invest in emerald. Today. In general, lighter and pinker skin tones are best flattered by colors with bluish undertones.

Universal Tip: *Any* great bag would work here; one that matches the outfit or is in bold contrast to it. The silver shoe is a neutral so go wild! Try a bag with rhinestones! Beads! Prints!

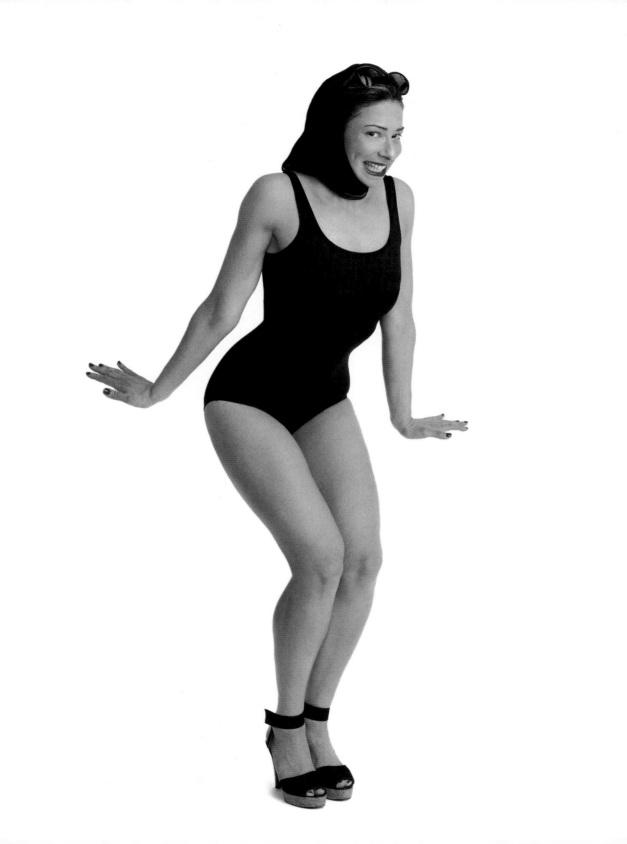

Curvy,
Average Height

STACY
5-foot-7
Size 4

"Being curvy or 'hourglass' has its ups and downs. Curves can be sexy but they can also make you look larger than you are if you don't dress them correctly. Super-low-cut jeans give me mean love handles! Sometimes I think it would be nice just to have a straight, stringbean body. You know, never worry about a bra, wear boy's jeans . . . Nobody really thinks of an hourglass as 'waifish.' Vampy, yes. Waifish, no. And vampy can cross into vulgar real fast if you're not careful. I think I'm at my happiest body-wise when I know I've chosen things that really walk that line of being professional and vaguely sexy at the same time."

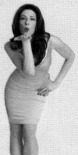

Clinton says I'm only 5-foot-6¾, but screw him.

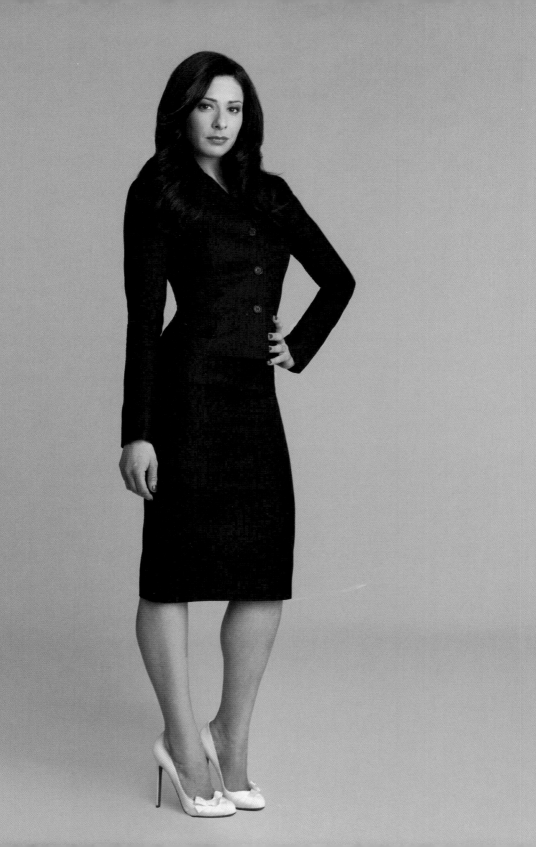

Curvy,
Average Height
Work

Let us say this about black for day: if you are going to do it, do it deliberately, not because you couldn't find anything to match that awful multicolor sweater that's been sitting in your drawer for a year. Black with primary colors tends to look dated. Don't fall back on black. It's not a safety net. It doesn't mean you have to wear black all by itself all the time, but rather than mixing it with brights, try other neutrals to accent it.

Black *is* slimming—when it's made by Dolce & Gabbana. It is the cut of clothing first and foremost that makes clothes slimming. If it doesn't fit, it isn't slimming. Then, consider that all darker colors camouflage while lighter colors emphasize.

A beautiful suit like this is formal enough to take you right from work into drinks and dinner.

With an hourglass figure, your chest and hips are already larger than your waist. Look for jackets that follow the natural line of your body, which narrow at the waist or either sit at the top of the hip or flare from the hip.

With a naturally short torso and long legs, the straight skirt can cover the knee, but going too much longer will make you look matronly. Without a super-high heel, you may want to go to the middle of the kneecap.

The best accessory for a fitted straight skirt suit is a structured bag with short handles or a clutch (or a riding crop).

Note from Stacy: Not everyone wears 4-inch heels to work, but that's part of my job. When you have to stand next to someone all day—every day, day after day—who's 9 inches taller, you may develop an addiction to a higher heel. (Clinton still hasn't agreed to pay for my podiatrist and chiropractic bills, but I'm working on it.)

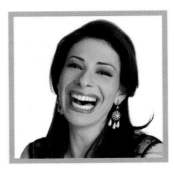

Color Palette

Choose an interesting yet related color palette when coordinating your jewelry. Here the necklace is turquoise, which pops on the teal top and dark blue denim. But other color combinations that work are burgundy with rose quartz, coral with orange, and cream with pearls.

Curvy,
Average Height
Weekend

A three-quarter topper coat is a good length for an average height (5-foot-4 to 5-foot-7). If you're shorter, it can be overwhelming. And if you're taller, it can look too small. But to keep a good line on the body, keep the coat open and go with a top that is short (to the waistline) and a midrise, narrow straight jean to look leggy.

Darker wash **jeans** have a tendency to look more sophisticated than lighter ones because they look more like trousers and can do double duty from day to night.

Finding cool tops when you have a chest and want to wear a supportive bra can be hard in a world full of spaghetti straps. (We're not big fans of showing the bra strap underneath.) Look for T-shirt shapes in fancier fabrics with more intricate detailing and nice V-neck lines instead of grabbing the nearest halter.

While we recommend jewelry that matches the stature of the person, you can use bolder necklaces (here in two lengths) to balance the length and light color of the **coat.**

Universal Tip: A white coat can be deadly. Wear it once and it looks gray by the time you get home. But a subtle print can hide a bit of the grime we encounter every day and is great for both spring and fall.

Universal Tip: When you find your favorite cut of jean, buy more than one pair. Have one hemmed to wear with high heels and the other with flats so your jeans are always the right length no matter what the occasion.

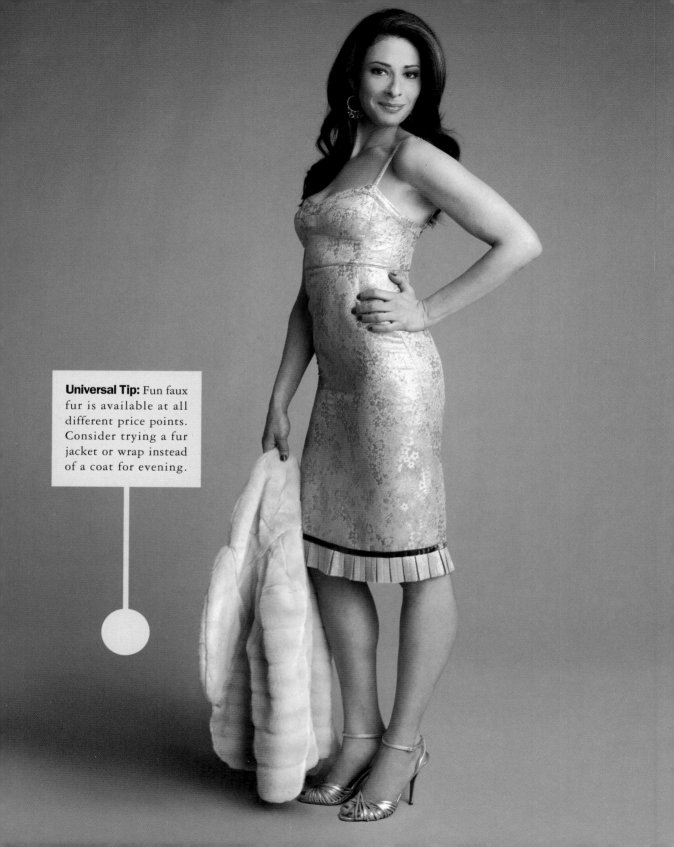

Universal Tip: Fun faux fur is available at all different price points. Consider trying a fur jacket or wrap instead of a coat for evening.

Curvy,
Average Height
Evening

Choose a straight dress for an hourglass shape to accentuate curves.

Spaghetti-strap dresses are tricky. You either need to wear a strapless bra or choose a dress that gives the Girls bra-like support. The straps should fit securely as they would on a bra, and the seaming should give lift and simulate the support of a cup. (Note from Stacy: Clinton is cringing right now, but, ladies, you need to know this.)

The pleated hem here is a contrasting color and different material that helps to balance the width of the hip.

Beware, however, when choosing a shiny fabric (this one is a **metallic** brocade); anywhere light hits will be emphasized like a spotlight on a stage. (Note from Stacy: I can't tell you how thrilled I am to have that spotlight on my thigh.)

An ankle strap on the heel works here, even for average height, because an empire waist makes your waistline look higher than it is naturally, therefore interrupting the length of the leg isn't as consequential.

Try mixing textures for a sophisticated evening look. If you are wearing a dress with a sheen to it, do a flat wrap or coat. Or vice-versa: wear a dress with no sheen and top it with a metallic brocade coat or one with lots of sparkly embellishment.

Hubba-hubba!

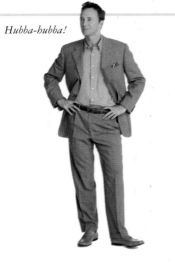

Universal Tip: Pale metallics work better on olive or dark skin. (Note from Clinton: Stacy's actually pretty pale, but thanks to a spray tan and her aspiration to be J-Lo, she wore this dress anyway.)

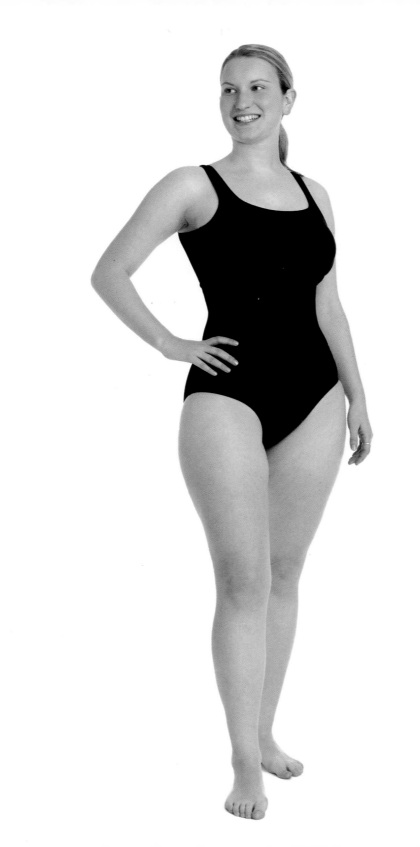

Curvy,
Tall

JESSICA
5-foot-10
Size 12

"My favorite body part is definitely my waist. Even when I gain weight, it is still defined and highlights my curves. I have a large chest and a small back, though, and it's hard for me to find dresses that fit well and with which I can wear a heavy-duty bra. My chest never seems to fit in anything properly."

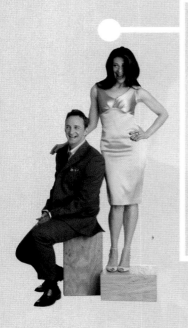

STACY AND CLINTON SAY: "Living with a larger chest can be hard sometimes. For most people when they gain weight, their shape remains the same. So hourglasses are more likely to gain weight in the chest and hips rather than the waist. With a large chest and a small back, avoid spaghetti straps or seams that create and 'hem in' a smaller bustline—anything that will make you look squished or unable to wear supportive foundational garments. Look for pieces and fabrics with give in them, like jersey. Jessica is fortunate in that she has hips to balance her chest, a really narrow waist, and thin limbs. And because she is tall, her body can easily look long and lean in all the right pieces."

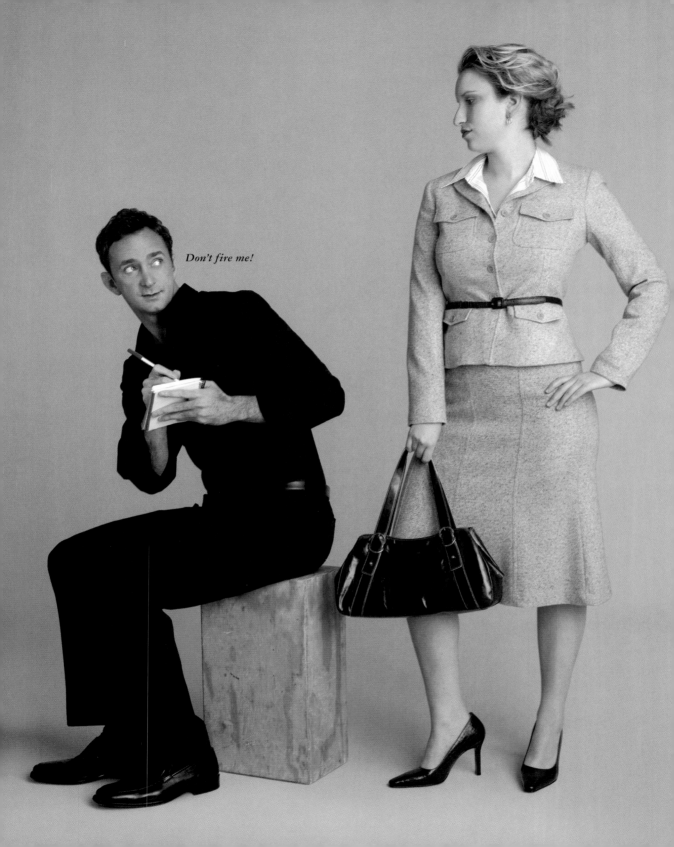

Don't fire me!

Curvy,
Tall
Work

A **pale** tweed is a real staple to think about when buying a suit. You can break it up with other pieces (think hot pink cashmere twin set with the skirt, and pale gold sequin tank and jeans with the jacket!) and it works well in both spring and fall.

Look for a paneled, slightly trumpet-flared skirt to accent the curve of the hip but to help de-emphasize a larger thigh. Make sure it falls past the knee if you are taller than 5-foot-9.

The short boxy blazer has multiple buttons for locking and loading a large chest and accenting a short torso.

By adding a belt on top of the jacket, you can call attention to a narrow waist and create a waist. If you have a little bit of a tummy, this trick can still work for you, contrary to what you might think: place the belt just above the natural waist where you are narrower. The belt becomes the focal point and the tummy is camouflaged by the flare in the jacket created by the cinch of the belt.

Hosiery Tip: Tweed looks great with a patterned tight, like argyle or herringbone. Just be sure the size of the pattern is in keeping with the size of your overall body.

Universal Tip: Like pale neutrals but afraid they will wash you out? Do a shot of color by the face in a prominent collared shirt or sweater.

Universal Tip: As we seem to always say, "Shoes and bags don't have to match, they have to go." But that doesn't mean they can't match. It's a matter of personal preference. We love mock croc—it's just leather that has been embossed to look like real crocodile skin. It can look so expensive and cost a fraction of the price!

Seasonal Alternative:
Too hot for boots? When you're tall, flat sandals are a great option. Also, wedge sandals look great with wrap dresses and give them a '70s vibe.

Do yourself a favor. Want to wear multi-tiered necklaces? Buy an all-in-one. Less tangle, less hassle. Only one to keep track of.

Curvy,
Tall
Weekend

A wrap dress is ideal for showing off curves if you've got 'em—and Jessica's got awesome curves. The wrap's just the best item to have in your closet for emphasizing a narrow midsection.

Look for a wrap that ties somewhere between the top of your rib cage and your natural waist, which is, in most cases, the most narrow part of the body.

The sash here is just below the breast and, almost like an empire seam, creates the appearance of a short torso and longer legs.

Most **wrap** dresses have a flattering V-shaped neckline. Choose one to show as much cleavage as you feel comfortable with. The deeper V here helps to balance a larger chest.

Think about proportion when looking for the perfect wrap dress: a thick sash like the one pictured here helps to balance Jessica's height and the shape of her curves. It's proportionate to Jessica's stature.

The same goes when looking for prints: match the size of the print to the size of the person. This all-over pattern doesn't overwhelm Jessica. On a smaller woman, it might.

A knee-high boot is perfect to wear with skirts and dresses when you are tall or have superlong legs. Petites take the risk of losing too much leg line by attempting the same look. Who wants to look like they are standing in a bucket? Stick to a lower boot, like midcalf height, if you're shorter.

A paler-color boot works here with the paleness of Jessica's dress and doesn't take away from her body shape and length. Her gams are covered but still look long and fabulous.

Universal Tip: Some wrap dresses are complicated to tie. (No joke! We know it's not brain surgery, but sometimes they can be a little tricky.) So look for faux wrap dresses that are sewn to look like they wrap but don't. All you usually have to do is pull one over your head.

*Matching cuff
or bangle
bracelets can
make an elegant
statement
for evening.*

Curvy,
Tall
Evening

Wearing a full-length dress is all about making an entrance. Doesn't Jessica remind you of a modern-day Grace Kelly? Full-length dresses make the most of height and curves.

Let us say a word about black for night: it doesn't go out of style. It is what we associate with evening dress. It isn't called black tie for nothing. Trends come and go. Color for evening is in, then it's out, then in, and so on. You can always pair a black dress with a brilliantly colored pair of shoes or a bright color bag (which we did here). But sometimes, just black—a black dress and shoe and bag—looks just perfect. It's timeless and classic. It works on all skin types, but we especially love it here on Jessica's pale skin and light hair.

The **diagonal** pattern of the tiers and the alternate use of satin and velvet on this gown accent Jessica's natural body shape but also create the optical illusion of narrowness.

With a deep-V neckline and "almost" cap sleeve, this dress still allows you to wear a supportive bra and show some cleavage.

The sleeve is set wide—almost *off* the shoulder—which maximizes the width of the shoulder and makes it proportionate with the width of the hip.

Larger jewelry is essential here to balance the impact of this dress. We chose a dramatic pair of chandelier earrings (a MUST-have in every woman's jewelry collection). But you could also do a necklace (or necklaces) with some impact. We caution trying to do both at the same time. Too much jewelry takes away from the outfit and the wearer herself. If your ears feel naked when you wear just a necklace, do a small stud so not everything is competing for attention on your head.

Some tall women fear the high heel. "I don't want to look taller than my date." We say, celebrate your height, even at the expense of your man's ego. If he's worth it, he'll get over it and worship you for the Amazonian goddess you are.

> **Universal Tip:** Look for dresses with angled tiers, stripe patterns, or seams in the shape of a V or upside-down V (called "chevron") to get this narrowing effect. Also, a raised hem on the front of a long dress ensures no stepping on the small train in back.

Not Curvy,
Overall

DON'T attempt to wear clothing that doesn't fit your chest or tush. You'll look like you are playing dress-up.

DO go for clingier clothes such as knitwear and boy-cut pants that help create curves.

MUST-HAVE: something supersexy! You can pull this off without being vulgar, so think halter top, backless dress, etc.

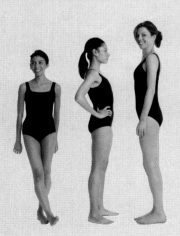

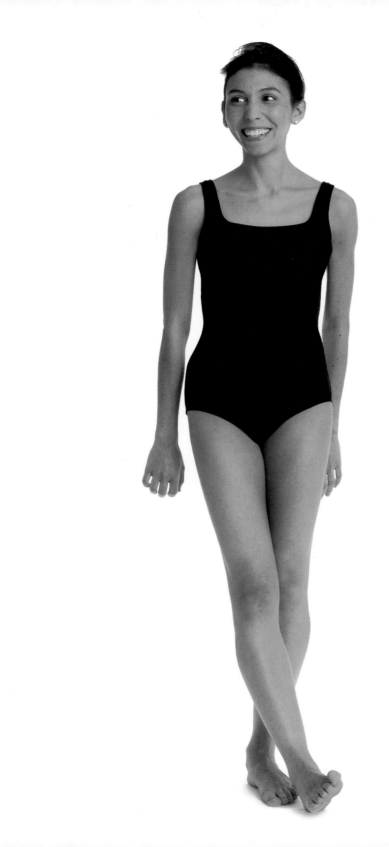

Not Curvy,
Petite

PARISE
5-foot-2
Size 0

"My biggest challenge is finding clothes to fit my petite frame. Everything is cut too big. I can just hold up an item and know that it will be baggy, so most of the time I don't even go through the effort of trying things on. Due to my size, people always think I'm younger than I am."

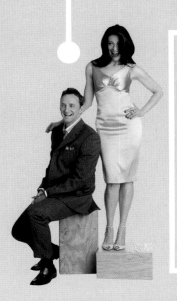

STACY AND CLINTON SAY: "Parise has the quintessential dancer's body and we sympathize with her plight in finding suitable sizes. She's so tiny, she could fit into kids clothes, but obviously that doesn't help Parise look like a professional, sexy woman. One of our first rules of thumb when dealing with small sizes is to look for European rather than American cuts. Europeans always cut smaller. So, we're looking for silhouettes that will give an impression of authority in the workplace, age-appropriateness on the weekend, and sophistication for evenings. And regardless of what Parise may think, you always have to try clothes on. You never know until you try. (Words to live by!)"

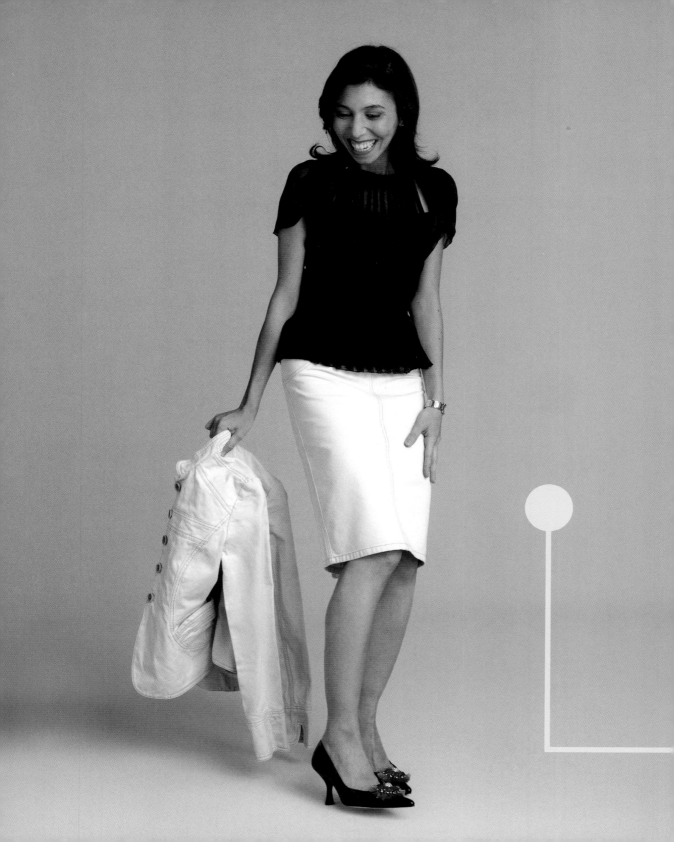

Not Curvy,
Petite
Work

A suit will always lend more of an authoritative air than separates, especially important for small-framed women in the workplace. It's easier to swallow orders from a woman in a suit than one in a plaid miniskirt.

Look for white and lighter colors to create more physical presence. (This is the opposite of "Black is slimming!") because the lighter the color, the more it reflects the light and the person wearing it.

Vertical pleating in a blouse can add the appearance of volume to the torso.

Look for cap sleeves to broaden the shoulder—they're helpful in creating a more womanly silhouette. If you have a curvier frame or larger arms, you may want to avoid this style so as not to create the illusion of *more* mass.

The seaming at the midsection of this blouse emphasizes the narrowness of the waist, while the peplum (the part that flares out beneath it) exaggerates the curve of the hip. More curves = grown-up!

Straight skirts create curves especially when they narrow at the hem by accenting the curve of the hip and thigh to the knee.

Don't go too high with the **heels.** Instead of looking sophisticated, you'll wind up looking like you raided your mom's closet. Anything that throws the petite frame out of proportion looks more like a costume than a stylish outfit.

Universal Tip: For a new twist on an old shoe, add shoe clips—they're like brooches for your shoes—and give them a second life!

Universal Tip: If you buy a suit, you can always break it up and use the parts with different pieces for new looks!

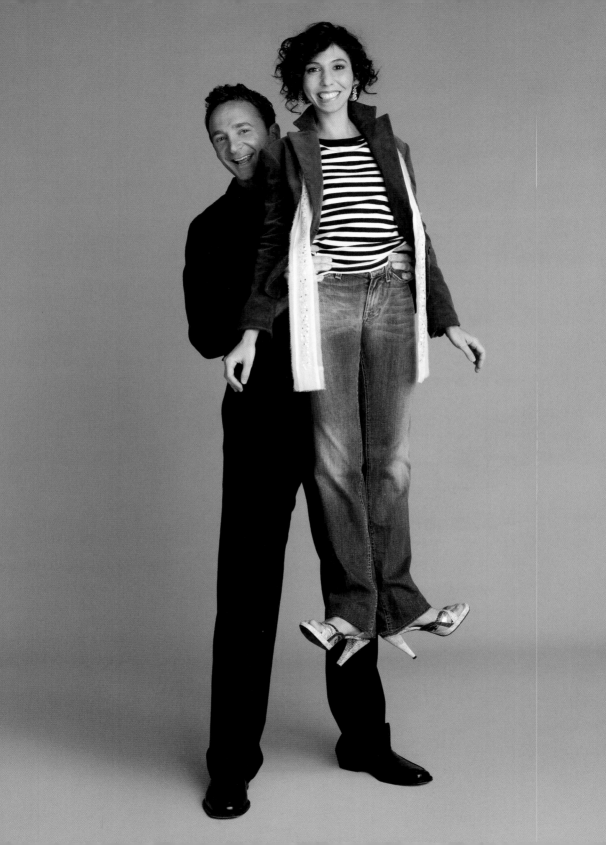

Not Curvy,
Petite
Weekend

First and foremost when dealing with a petite frame, finding the perfect fit is essential. Clothes that look too big will look like you borrowed them from your older sister. And clothes that are too small or show too much skin will make you look like a teenybopper. While we recommend a fitted blazer for almost everyone, this item is particularly important for those looking for a more sophisticated style. The inherent structure of a **blazer** is authoritative and always fashionable.

Knitwear creates more bulk than broadcloth shirting and is easier to fit on petites, as it clings and tends to come in smaller sizes.

Horizontal stripes create the appearance of a broader frame by forcing the eye sideways as opposed to up and down.

Jeans with bleaching or whiskering (those artificially created "wrinkles" around the crotch and the top of the thigh) also create emphasis on hips and thighs by calling attention to them.

Sophisticated accessories like metallic snakeskin sandals, a silk scarf with embellishment, and chandelier earrings can "grow up" an outfit without making the wearer look *too* old.

We know we were trying to make Parise look "less petite," but Clinton just couldn't keep from literally sweeping this cutie right off her feet.

Universal Tip: Casual blazers don't have to be in just neutral colors to get the maximum use out of them. This one is a leaf green, which falls into the category of what we call "pseudo-neutrals"—colors like the usual crop of neutrals (navy, black, gray, tan) that you can pair with just about any other color. Some other pseudo-neutrals: burgundy, army green, and light blue to name a few.

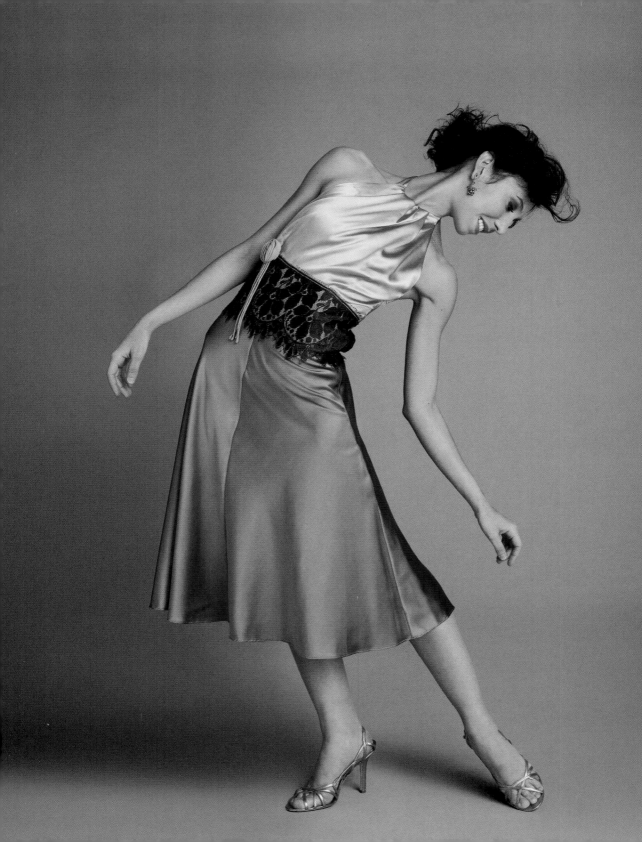

Not Curvy,
Petite
Evening

Use fabrics with sheen, especially silk charmeuse, to call attention to body shape. (Use with caution if you want to deemphasize a body area!)

The lace inset on this dress calls attention to and creates a narrow waistline.

Look for halter tops to emphasize the shoulder, creating a broader silhouette.

Softly draped A-line skirts add volume to a straight frame.

The straighter the frame, the longer the body looks naturally, so skirt lengths can be a little longer than for other petite body types.

A **tricolor** construction gives each body part (top, waist, and legs) its own emphasis and therefore a longer silhouette.

Now that's sheer elegance!

Universal Tip: Look for innovative color palettes. They look more sophisticated than primary colors. Imagine what a different impact this dress would have in red, blue, and yellow. We'd have a circus act instead of a cocktail dress.

Universal Tip: Oodles of accessories are unnecessary when there is so much going on in the dress. A small drop earring doesn't compete with the beauty of bare arms and legs.

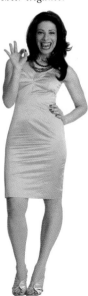

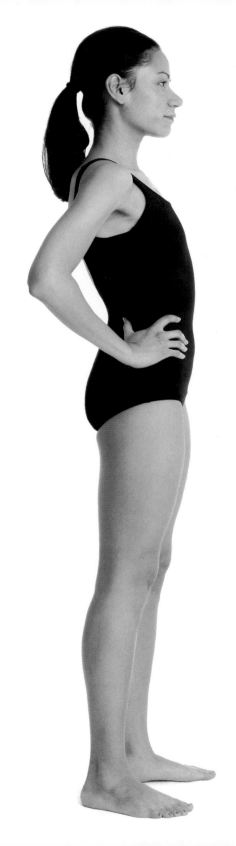

Not Curvy,
Average Height

JESSICA
5-foot-4
Size 2/4

"I love my flat stomach. I work on it every day. I have a very small bust, and so finding shirts that fit is pretty difficult, but I have pretty broad shoulders, which also makes fit tricky."

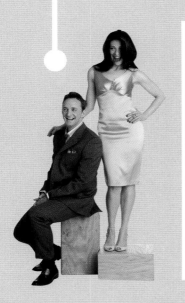

STACY AND CLINTON SAY: "Look for knitwear or materials mixed with stretch fabrics that will cling to the body. When you have defined shoulders and a small chest, it's hard to find nonstretch fabrics that will fit in both areas. Jessica is superlean and because of that looks much taller than she is. We want to emphasize that sense of height but play on her natural proportions to give her some curves. Even though she is average height, being so straight can also be difficult for giving her a more adult look. Jessica is proud of her waistline so we want to find clothing that will accentuate that and show off the parts of her body she likes the most."

Our Top Five Favorite Color Combos for Work
- Brown and pink
- Navy and lavender
- Brown, gray, and green
- Camel and orange
- Black, camel, and red

Not Curvy,
Average Height
Work

The bright pink piping on this suit is like a highlighter that draws curves in. The rounded vertical seam on the jacket gives her the appearance of a larger bustline, while the horizontal seaming at the midsection defines her narrow waist.

The vertical seamsn the skirt keep her looking long and the panels those seams create add volume and curve to her straight frame.

Look for fitted blazers with this kind of seaming, even if you don't like a bright contrasting-color piping. It is the seaming that creates tthe shape; the **color** just makes it more noticeable.

Remember, fitted shoulders and a narrow, nipped-in waist make this a good jacket for adding curves.

The trumpet skirt adds volume to the lower half without adding bulk. Jessica doesn't look bigger; she looks curvier.

We always say the great thing about a suit is that you can break up the pieces and wear them separately to create new outfits. In this case, both the jacket and the skirt individually help to create a curvier figure. The jacket paired with a long straight jean would add volume at the hip. And a fitted V-neck sweater with this skirt would define a sexy silhouette.

This suit was tailor-made for a body like Jessica's!

Universal Tip: Brown and pink. We love this color combo for day. *Très chic.*

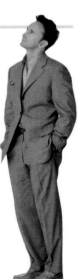

For cooler weather, try a turtleneck instead of the cotton broadcloth shirt you see here. Instead of a lightweight ("summer") denim, look for a heavier one. Or try a fitted corduroy jacket for the same effect.

Hem your pants so they sit on the top of your shoe; never let them touch the bottom of the heel . . . skim it, about a half-inch from the ground.

Not Curvy,
Average Height
Weekend

To give the illusion of some more curves on a straight body, go for a stretch denim jacket that fits closely to the body with midwaist seaming or stitching. It helps to define the waist and flares to create a curvature of the hip. (This jacket could also look great with a circle skirt and wedge heels for the weekend or a lighter tweed pencil skirt with sling-backs for work!)

When you have a small chest (or tush, for that matter!), look for pockets with a flap or larger buttons or snaps. The three-dimensional aspect of the pocket will highlight the area and give it a bit more . . . oomph. (Conversely, if you have a large chest or derrière, stay away from this kind of pocket detailing and stick with flat, seamed pockets. New styles include slightly angled pockets that can make the body-surface area appear smaller!)

Try wearing boy-cut (they have a very square cut at the hip), lower-rise trousers to put emphasis on hips, tush, and thighs. They highlight curves on even the straightest of female frames.

Think about the materials you wear when dressing the straight frame. Thicker or slightly stiffer corduroy or denim emphasizes the frame without making the body look unnatural.

A large collar and cuff call attention to the top half where more curves are highlighted by the cut of the jacket.

A squarer toe on the shoe works here. It's appropriate for this casual outfit and Jessica's legs are so lean, they aren't truncated by a shorter toe box.

A Word About Cut for the Straighter Frame: We know it seems nonsensical, but the best way to create curves on a straight frame is to find the tightest fit (without being constricting) in the most boyish cut. Strangely, we haven't seen this work on any guys we know, but this just proves our point that different cuts of clothing do different things for different body types.

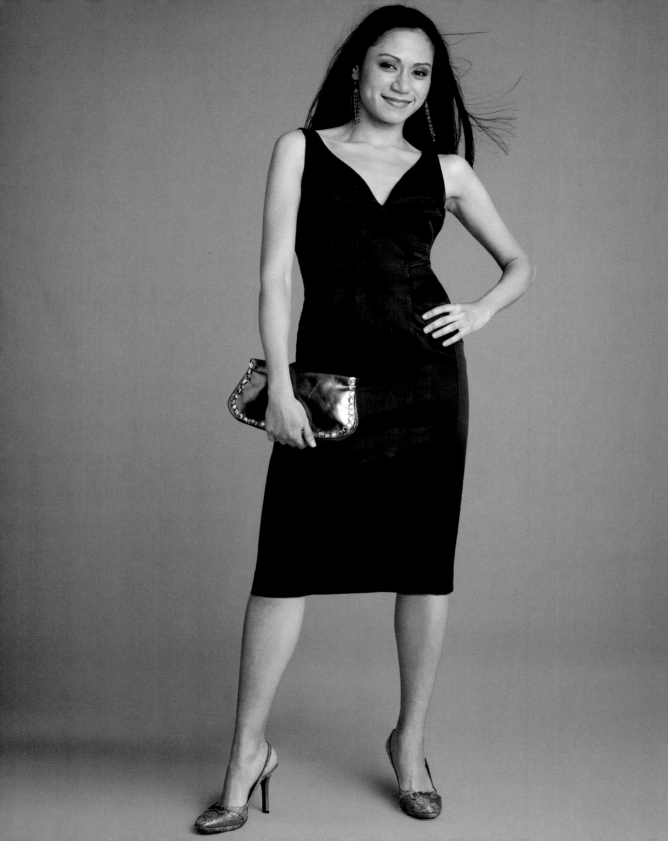

Not Curvy,
Average Height
Evening

Jessica was surprised by how much she liked this dress. She didn't think brown would look appropriate for evening. *Au contraire* . . . (That's French for "Not so fast, buster . . .")

The chocolate color on Jessica's olive skin (especially when paired with metallic accessories) is a super combination. Deep brown works on pale complexions as well. It's not quite as harsh as black (even grays can be), which have much colder undertones. Brown is a warm hue that echoes the tones in olive skin while warming up paler skin.

Look for a deep V in the front of a dress like this or even something backless to show off skin (which is always sexy) and highlights the area exposed.

Try a pencil dress made of a stretch satin fabric to hug the body and create the illusion of more curves.

As with the suit Jessica wore, the most important feature here is the seaming. All that stitching creates panels of emphasis in different parts of the body, and the sheen of the dress highlights those areas even more. Note the empire seaming to emphasize the bustline. There's an almost diamond-shaped front panel at the midsection that features a waistline. And the vertical side seams highlight the curve of the hip.

Skirt lengths to the knee are most flattering, balancing Jessica's height.

A rounded-toe metallic-brocade sling-back is fine here. Again, when you are average height and super straight, the need to elongate the leg is not as important as when you are trying to balance a curvier body. But high heels are always sexy for evening.

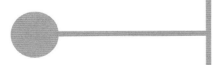

Shine Alert! Note that Jessica's dress, bag, and shoes all have a sheen to them. Vary the degree of shine between items in an outfit. People should admire your style, not be blinded by it!

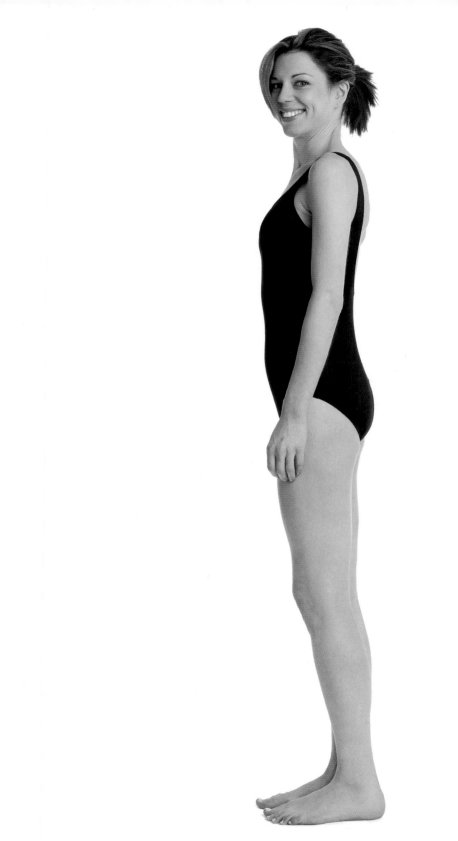

Not Curvy,
Tall

JANICE
5-foot-10
Size 4/6

"My biggest frustration is that jeans and pants are never long enough. Regardless, my favorite body part are my legs. They're long and strong. I wear a lot of tank tops because they seem to fit me best."

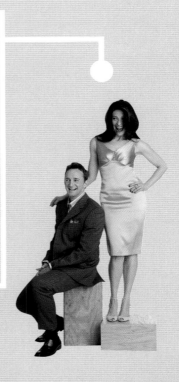

STACY AND CLINTON SAY: "We know. We know. Tall women are forever begging us to help them find long pants. It's a pain to find them, but they're out there. Because longer trousers became all the rage a few years back, the selection is growing. We prefer a men's-style trouser when you're tall with a willowy frame to help balance your height with a little bit of width. Like every body type, there are pros and cons to having it. While most women would kill to be tall and superlean, the women who do actually have this body worry about appearing gawky and looking like they outgrew their clothes when sleeves aren't long enough and the hem of a pant leg is just too short. This frame, in particular, benefits greatly from layering and adding a bit of volume to the limbs. We are going for statuesque here, people, not awkward."

Suit Schmoot

While the successful (or even hoping-to-be-successful) woman needs at least one killer suit in her wardrobe, she also needs a few other wardrobe staples. Here are our top five. Hmmm . . . we smell a quiz coming. Got all five already? You're executive material. Got three or four? You're ready to climb the corporate ladder. One or two? It's entry-level only, babe. Got none? How does life in the mailroom sound?

• A fitted turtleneck
• A fitted A-line skirt
• A silk blouse
• A fitted jacket
• A classic trench—which would look awesome, by the way, with Janice's outfit here!

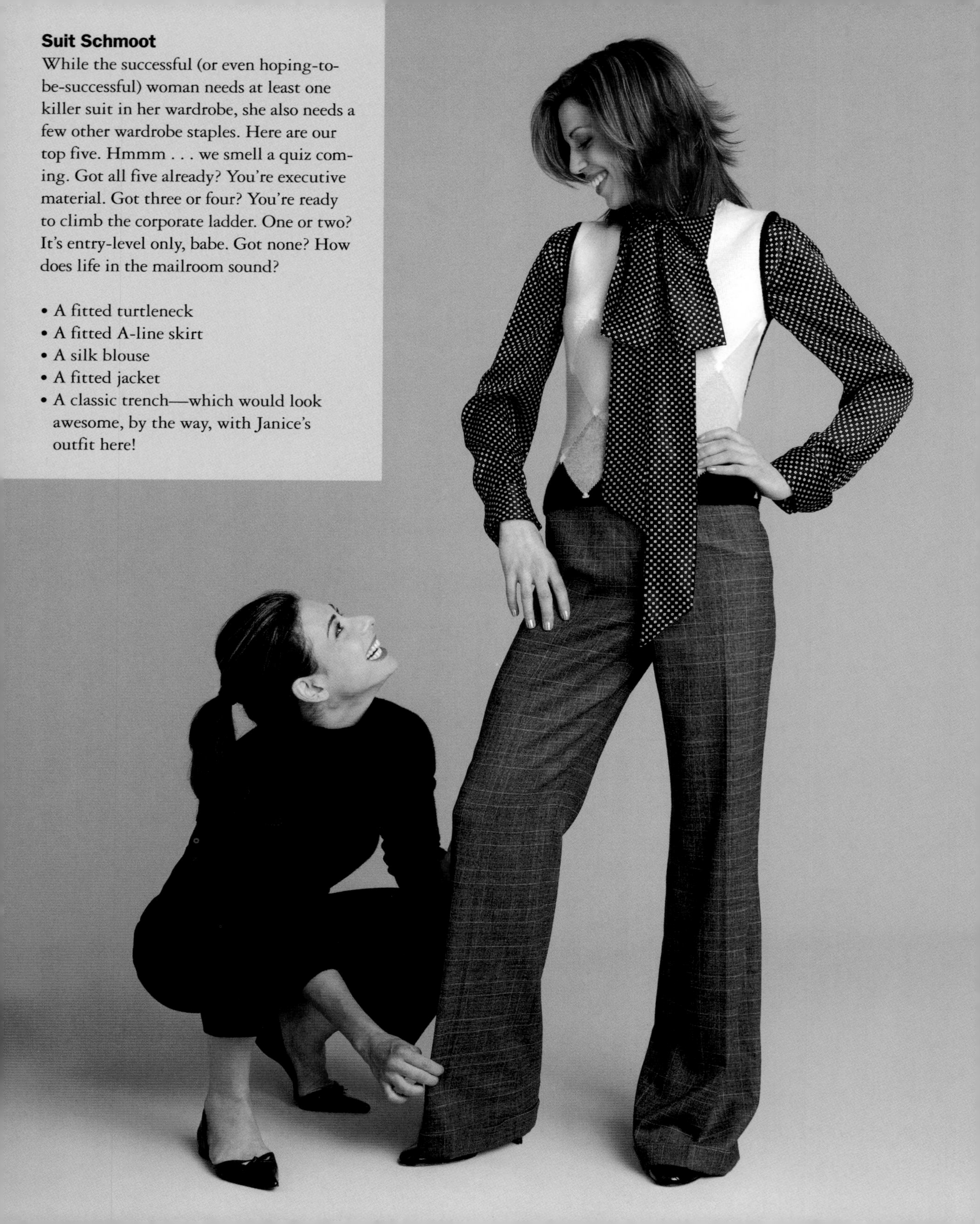

Not Curvy,
Tall
Work

We loved this outfit on Janice. She reminded us of all the fabulous ladies who pioneered the pant look: Kate Hepburn, Marlene Dietrich, Greta Garbo.

As we've said, adding a little bit of volume with billowy fabrics can create an attractive silhouette for this body type. Look for a trouser that has a men's cut to it. Here, a tropical (that's a lighter weight, three-season) wool in a subtle glen plaid print is terrific for the width of the leg. It's slouchy, not sloppy, and adds a bit of volume to thin legs.

Normally, we think a cuff on a pant is a matter of taste, but when you are tall and thin, a cuff makes the pant look a bit heavier and adds more weight to the entire body shape. (If you are under 5-foot-4, cuffs just shorten the leg line, so steer clear of them.)

A bold, billowy blouse, like this silk polka-dot one with attached neck scarf, adds to a lean frame by having a slightly wider sleeve and the three-dimensional volume of the scarf itself. (A note about proportion: the scarf here is wide and long because Janice is so tall—and looks even taller with a straight frame—but adjust the size of the scarf to the size of the person. We don't want you looking like you've been strangled and swallowed by a piece of fabric.)

Layering is key to creating a fuller shape. Add a knit **vest** on top of the blouse to layer without bulk and to define a waistline. Here, the vest gets darker as it gets closer to the waist, adding even more attention to it.

Rounded-toe shoes look terrifically chic with this wider pant (maybe it's the '40s feel) and actually serve to keep the leg from looking too long.

Universal Tip: It's fine to mix patterns as long as they aren't all competing for attention. The argyle of this vest is the most prominent print while the glen plaid of the pant and the polka-dot of the blouse are just supporting players.

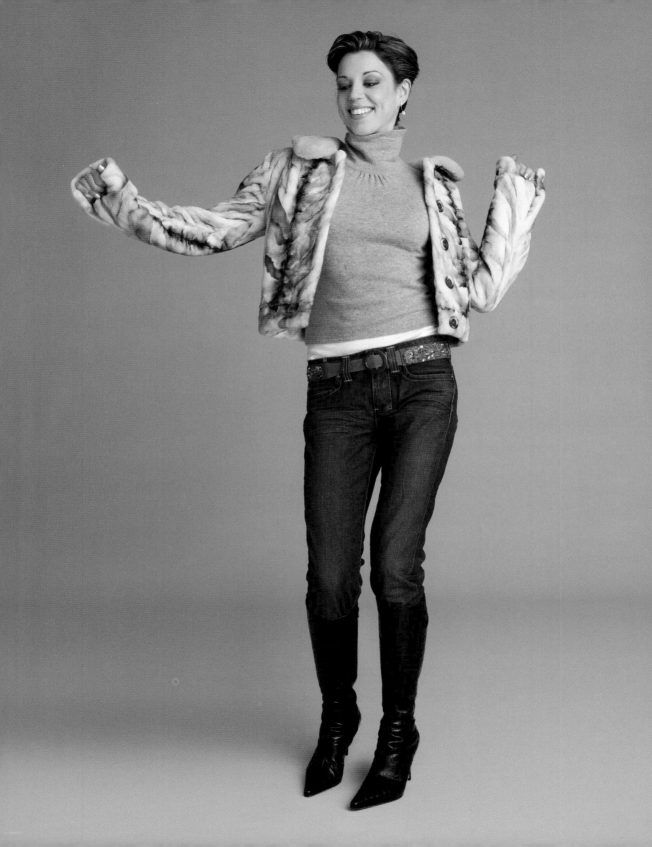

Not Curvy,
Tall
Weekend

Layering well to balance a lean frame is not the same as bulking up. We do not want you wearing layer after layer of oversized sweatshirts or Cosby sweaters to make your frame fuller. The idea here is to layer subtly, with fitted pieces, to create a balanced look with your height.

Look for boxy jackets (a.k.a. "chubbies") with a heavy fabric like fur or faux fur to broaden the torso and give a stronger shoulder impression. A big collar helps too.

Start with a longer-length long-sleeve T-shirt in a brighter tone, and top with a fitted shorter sweater. The hem of the tee will pop at the waistline, adding depth to an outfit and helping fill out the shape of the sweater.

Fitted turtlenecks make necks look less giraffe-like. On a tall, lean frame, the neck is like the limbs; you want to keep them looking graceful, not gawky.

Use heavier belts to emphasize a waist, especially ones with eye-catching interest, like beading or sequins.

Janice couldn't believe that we found jeans long enough for her, and even though you can't see the hem in the picture, we swear we did! Several different companies are now making special styles for the longer limbed, and a few make only these styles.

When your jeans aren't long enough but you love the way they fit, tuck them in as we have here. With a pointy **boot,** you shorten the body only slightly, which actually helps the proportion of a tall, thin frame.

Universal Tip: If your calves are so thin that you have trouble finding boots that fit, look for high boots made of stretch leather (yes, they make that now!) so that the boot clings to your leg.

Seasonal Alternative: For a more casual spring look, try some cool (read: *not athletic*) sneakers in a bright color. And switch out the chubby jacket for something that is still boxy but less heavy, like a summer-weight leather motorcycle jacket.

Tight clothes aren't the only way to attract attention. Clothing with volume looks fab on the dance floor. Skirts or dresses with major twirl factor show skin in flashes and have historically aided women in hooking a hottie. (It's true! How do you think Ginger Rogers snagged Fred Astaire?)

Not Curvy,
Tall
Evening

One way to create curves and a fuller frame for the straight body type is by wearing very fitted, straight pieces. The other way is to pair fitted pieces with pieces that actually have lots of volume. Especially when you have height to balance it, you can handle bigger pieces without looking overpowered.

Look for voluminous, full skirts to make the body appear more feminine.

Pair them with tanks that are fitted with a thicker rib and a deep scoop neckline. Wide-set thicker straps will be proportionate with a full skirt.

Make sure that the skirt length is well past your knee, even as long as the middle of the calf; otherwise this outfit looks less like something you'd wear to the ballet than like something in the ballet.

An ankle-strap sandal balances the width of the skirt and adds proportion overall to the frame of the body.

When wearing something as simple as a tank for evening, you may want to dress it up with a bold piece of **jewelry.** Be careful to make sure it's in balance with the print of the skirt and not competing with it. This necklace is a larger pendant, but still clean in its design and not overly fussy. Multilength chains here would be distracting.

Universal Tip: Embellishment (beading, sequins, rhinestones—sparkly bits) on clothing has been very popular the last few seasons. For day as well as evening. Whether it remains in or goes out of style is anyone's guess, but we feel a couple of embellished pieces for evening are a staple of any woman's wardrobe. They're always useful for a little "bling" and quite often negate the necessity for additional jewelry.

Extra Curvy,
Overall

DON'T go for too much ruffle and frill. While some embellishment on clothing is nice, don't go for things that add weight to the look of your frame. No loosey-goosey drapy fabrics; they have no shape and neither will you!

DO look for clothing with clean lines and flattering seaming. Look for stiffer fabrics that have structure.

MUST-HAVE: A structured leather or other stiff material jacket that sits at the top of the hip.

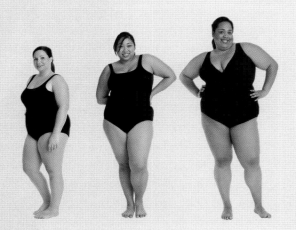

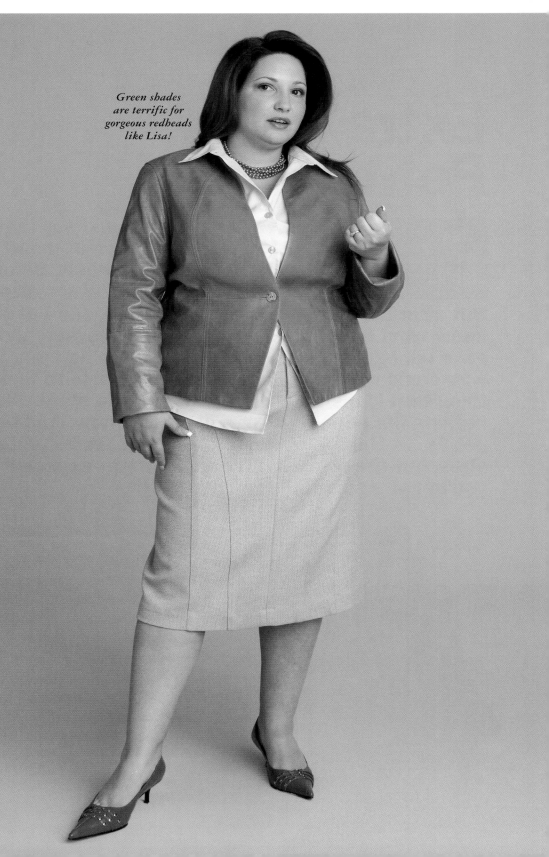

*Green shades
are terrific for
gorgeous redheads
like Lisa!*

Extra Curvy,
Petite
Work

The goal here is to play up the bust a little and play down the tummy. So, a single-button leather blazer creates a waistline by nipping in on the sides and creating a more hourglass shape. The jacket creates a strong V shape from the neckline down to the button closure and an inverse V from the hem of the jacket up to the button closure. A V shape at both the top and the bottom of the jacket creates a narrowing effect.

Usually, when you're petite, we recommend that you keep your skirts to the knee. However, here you want to keep the skirt longer, just below the knee, to keep in proportion with both the size of the bust and the waist.

A pointy shoe always helps to lengthen the leg, but avoid any kind of ankle strap, which would break the line of the leg.

Heavier-weight fabrics, like leather, help you control your body's shape better than flimsier ones—they have more structure. But keep in mind that you don't want to add bulk, so fit is everything. The shoulder seam is the most important for getting the jacket to fit correctly. Many plus-size women find that they cannot close a jacket that fits well in the shoulder. Buy only the jacket that closes and have the shoulder reset. This is not an inexpensive alteration but a priceless one. Your clothes will fit infinitely better.

Button-front shirts that have Lycra added will help you feel less constricted. The collar needs to lie flat, so we don't lose your neck.

The curved seams on this skirt help elongate the body and play up a womanly shape.

Universal Tip: We love khaki with bright color for day—instead of black!

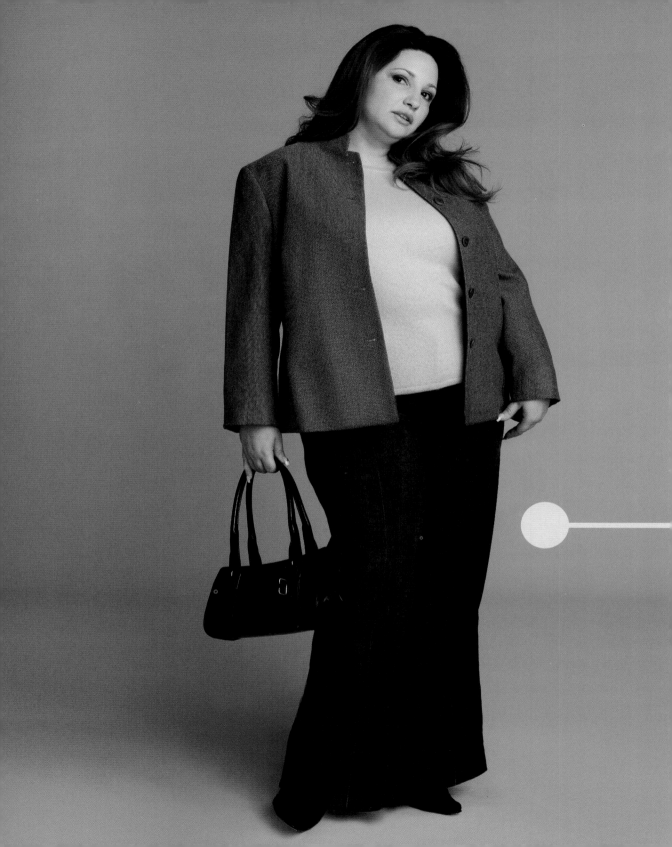

Extra Curvy,
Petite
Weekend

Boxier, shorter jackets that sit on top of the hip will help elongate the leg and give the impression of a narrower midsection.

We loved this shape on Lisa, but beware a Nehru collar—when it is closed, you can lose your neck completely.

A wider-leg jean helps balance the body. Just be sure to buy a straight leg, not a boot cut, which would emphasize the thigh and shorten the leg.

Small shoulder pads—not the linebacker or Linda Evans in *Dynasty* type—can help balance out a large chest and tummy.

A pointy boot, just like a pointy-toed shoe, elongates the line of the leg.

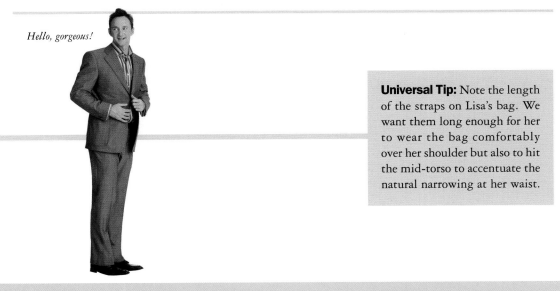

Hello, gorgeous!

Universal Tip: Note the length of the straps on Lisa's bag. We want them long enough for her to wear the bag comfortably over her shoulder but also to hit the mid-torso to accentuate the natural narrowing at her waist.

A Word About Color: We purposely put Lisa in these softer neutrals to give her weekend look a fresher sophistication and to highlight her peaches-and-cream skin tone and bronze hair color. The majority of plus-size clothing tends to be available in primary and pastel colors and a lot of black—all of which on their own can make a woman look matronly. Search for new ways to mix and match these colors, such as with softer neutrals or denim, to keep you stylish and current.

A note from Clinton: Lisa's my best friend from high school. I'm not kissing a complete stranger.

Extra Curvy,
Petite
Evening

You should never feel limited to dresses for evening. Separates can look just as sophisticated for evening, and they often fit a lot better!

Pleating under the bust of the camisole suggests a waistline without cinching. Look for clothes that create the hourglass shape without pulling too tightly on the body.

Lace detailing in a contrasting color on the sleeveless V-neck shell pulls attention toward the face.

A handkerchief hem (meaning an uneven hem) on a skirt provides wonderful movement, which calls attention to the narrowness of the lower leg.

A **shawl** is a great, dramatic accessory and provides some arm coverage. Just be careful that you choose the size of your shawl and the size of its print wisely. Anything too large will overwhelm an outfit and swallow you up. Remember, the idea is to accent the outfit with some style punch and camouflage anything you feel needs a bit a more coverage. Overdoing it is akin to wearing a sleeping bag for a night out on the town.

Hosiery Option: Because Lisa has a darker shawl on top, a black sheer stocking could work here, even one with a back seam or some sheen, without shortening the line of her leg and maintaining the sexiness of the look.

Universal Tip: Only have a few pieces you like to wear for evening? Make sure they fit as well as possible. Then change them up with fun accessories, like shawls and wraps, vintage costume jewelry, and fabulous shoes!

Seasonal Alternative: Just too cool for a silk shell, even with a wrap? Try a jacket with some sheen or a twin set with some embellishment (i.e., sequins, rhinestones, beads, etc.) for a look that provides more warmth but also structure and shape to an outft. Just stay away from any knitwear that is too clingy or heavily ribbed at the waistline.

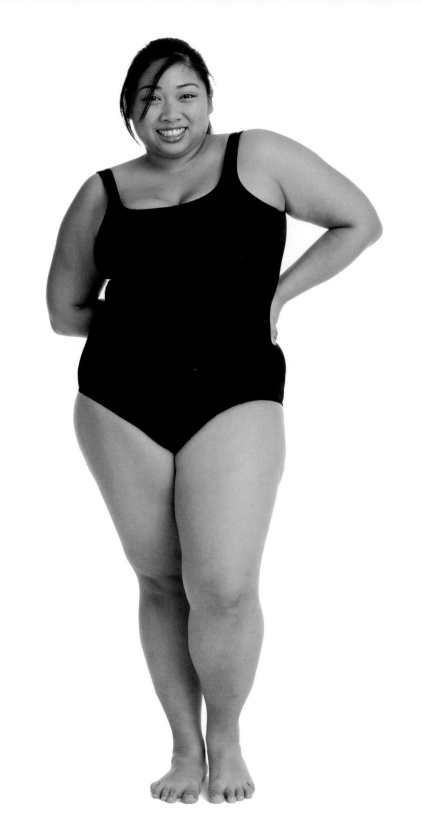

Extra Curvy,
Average Height

JULIE
5-foot-6
Size 20

"I love the way my chest and hips are both full and feminine. One day when I was on vacation in Trinidad, a man yelled out that I was 'thick like mud.' I think it was supposed to be a compliment. From the way he was smiling, that's how it felt. It is hard to find clothes that fit well on top. I hate wearing anything that looks baggy, but I don't want to look squeezed into something, either. It's difficult to buy larger clothes that are not circus tents or skanky."

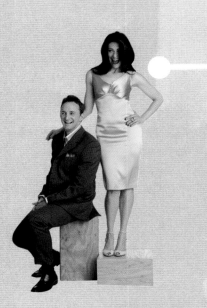

STACY AND CLINTON SAY: "We hear you, Julie. But the plus-size market is growing in leaps and bounds, just not as quickly as we'd like. Being comfortable with your body and liking it is so important but when you can't find clothes that fit it the way you'd like, it can get frustrating fast. We feel it's important to look for clean lines without tons of intricate detailing to keep the focus on the woman, not on the woman who is trying to hide in her clothes. We want to find more structured pieces for Julie—that fit her comfortably but don't look oversized—and keep her out of superfrilly items and in more architectural-looking pieces."

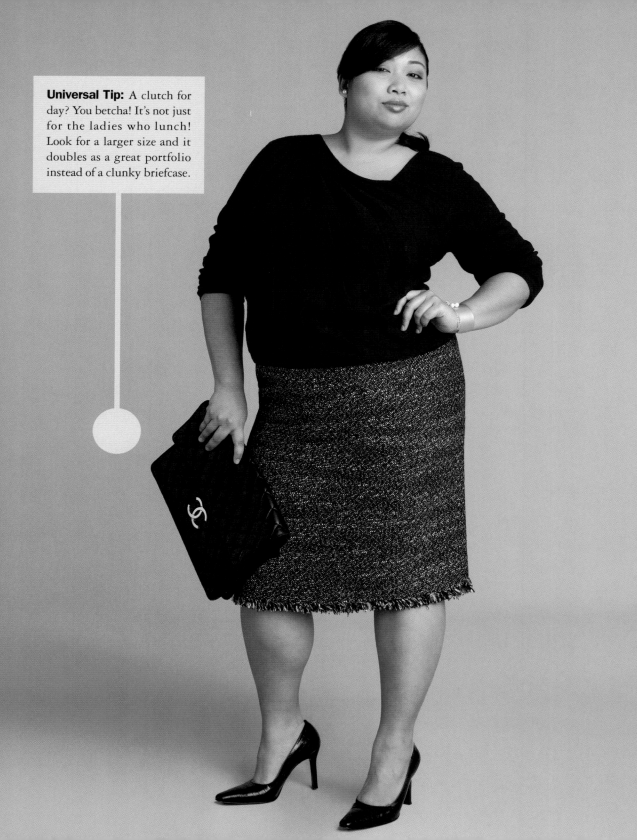

Universal Tip: A clutch for day? You betcha! It's not just for the ladies who lunch! Look for a larger size and it doubles as a great portfolio instead of a clunky briefcase.

Extra Curvy,
Average Height
Work

Sometimes the best thing to do is to keep things as simple as possible, especially when you're as well proportioned as Julie.

Pieces that fit well and closer to the body are ideal for plus sizes. Too much volume can add bulk to the frame. A well-fitting sweater and pencil skirt looked so great on Julie because she isn't hiding her shape.

Look for knits with necklines that don't "choke" away your neck and that fit comfortably in the arm and torso.

Note the asymmetric wave of the rib in the sweater. It flatters the torso more than a straight vertical rib would and adds an interesting visual detail.

A straight skirt that does not narrow at the knee plays up existing curves without exaggerating them.

By wearing a dark solid on top and a textured skirt on the bottom, you create a waistline where the two meet.

A word about tweed: be careful when purchasing this fabric in a plus size. It can create bulk. Look for thin-weight tweed or tweed with a thin lining so that it lies flat on the body and doesn't bunch up.

A woman's accessories should generally be in keeping with her stature. That's why this larger clutch works so well. The same goes for the cuff bracelet. Julie's a bigger girl—she says it her-self—and she shouldn't feel the need to apologize for that by wearing teensy-weensy jewelry.

Hosiery option: Julie has a few choices here. She could easily wear a textured, opaque tight with this look. To pop it into evening, however, she could try a black sheer stocking with a seam! *Woo-hoo!* Sexy!

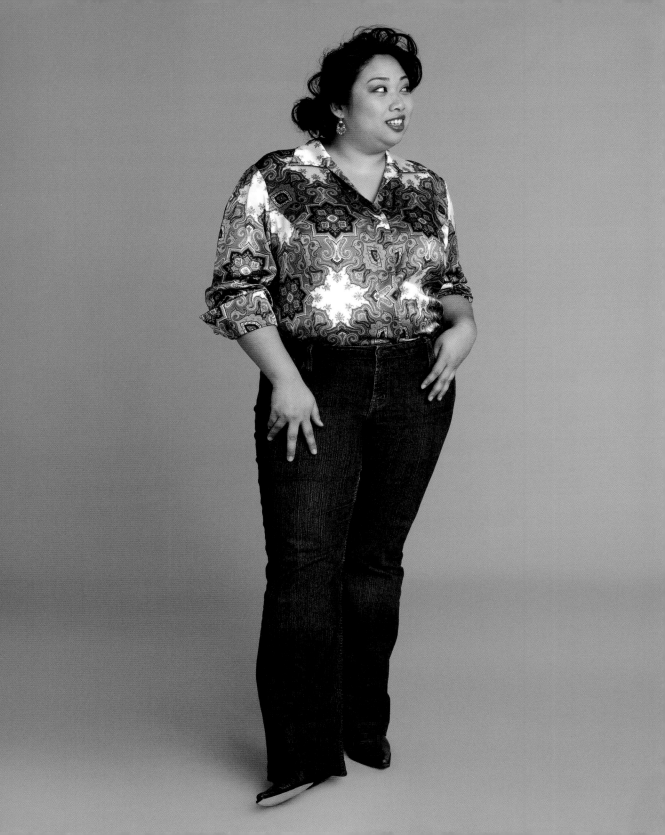

Extra Curvy,
Average Height
Weekend

A patterned shirt keeps the eye focused on the top half of the body, and the size of the pattern is proportionate to the size of the woman.

Boot-cut jeans can play up sexy curves *only* if you are well proportioned throughout the leg and you have some height to work with.

The pointy-toed cowboy boot, a heavier shoe than a dainty stiletto, is in keeping with Julie's frame and helps elongate the leg.

Belt Options: For a more casual look, forgo a belt altogether or select a thick or studded leather belt, with a big buckle to balance it. To dress your denim up a bit, look for a multi-chain-link belt that drapes below the loops; wear it to the side to give the appearance of a narrower waistline.

Try adding a tweed blazer over a silk printed blouse for a great "going out to brunch" look. The mix of texture and a bold pattern isn't overpowering. It looks cleverly creative.

Universal Tip: If you're going to do boot cut, make sure it fits you well in the thigh and that it has a uniform wash. Otherwise it can cause your thighs to look bigger and your legs shorter.

Seasonal Alternative: When adding a coat to a frame like Julie's, keep two things in mind: one, you don't want materials that will add bulk to the frame, and two, go for some length if you've got some height.
• Colder-weather fabrics can be bulky. Make sure when looking at wool coats that they have a full lining in a fabric that doesn't allow them to bulk up on the body.
• Always give yourself a little bit of extra room in a coat that you will wear only outdoors *over* outfits.
• You could easily add a great cashmere V-neck sweater to this look before topping it with a longer winter coat. Not only does smart layering keep you warm, it gives an outfit some depth and a look more put together.

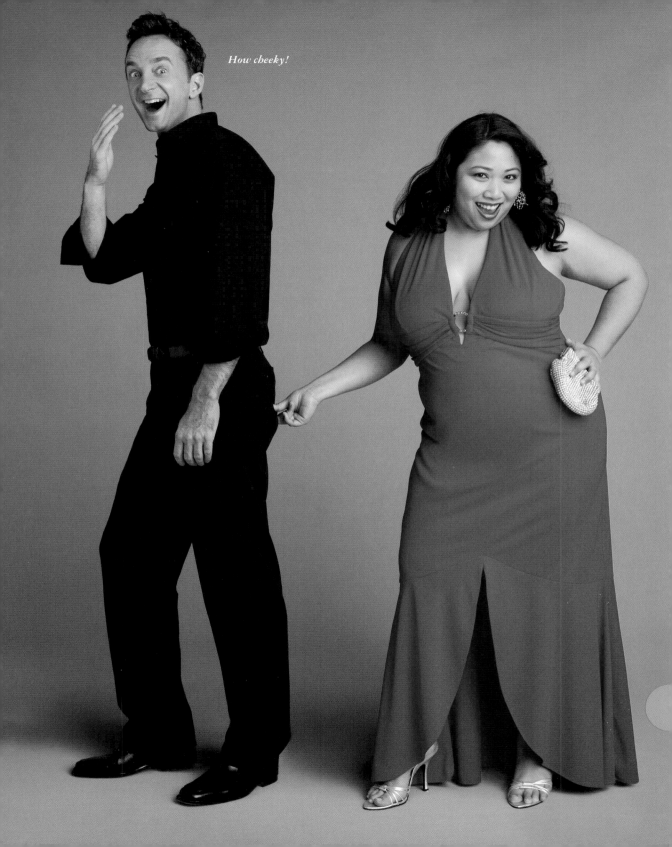

How cheeky!

Extra Curvy, Average Height
Evening

Julie looked so amazing in **red,** we told her she should wear it at least once a week. This kind of old-school glamour reminded us of Jayne Mansfield!

The deep-V neckline of this halter puts visual emphasis on the face and bustline while the extra ruching keeps the bust supported.

A convertible bra is essential for proper support when wearing a halter dress. Look for a deep-V bra with a front clear strap and detachable straps that can be reattached in a halter-strap configuration.

The neckline echoes the front slit of the dress, creating a vertical illusion of a longer frame. At 5-foot-6, Julie is tall, but the cut of this dress makes her look even longer.

The seam that angles upward just above the knee also creates this sense of length by creating the illusion of a longer leg line.

Please don't try to wear a coat the same length as a full-length dress. It's just too overwhelming on any frame. Try a fabulous wrap to keep the glam factor high!

Fresh!

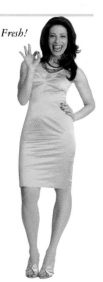

Universal Tip: We love red with silver as opposed to red and gold. The latter combo can look a little too much like a Christmas ornament. An alternative to metallic accessories would be another bright color; accents of violet or light blue look spectacular with a red dress like this!

Universal Tip: Full-length dresses are for formal occasions—black-tie galas and red-carpet events. Be sure to wear this appropriately. It's not for cocktails.

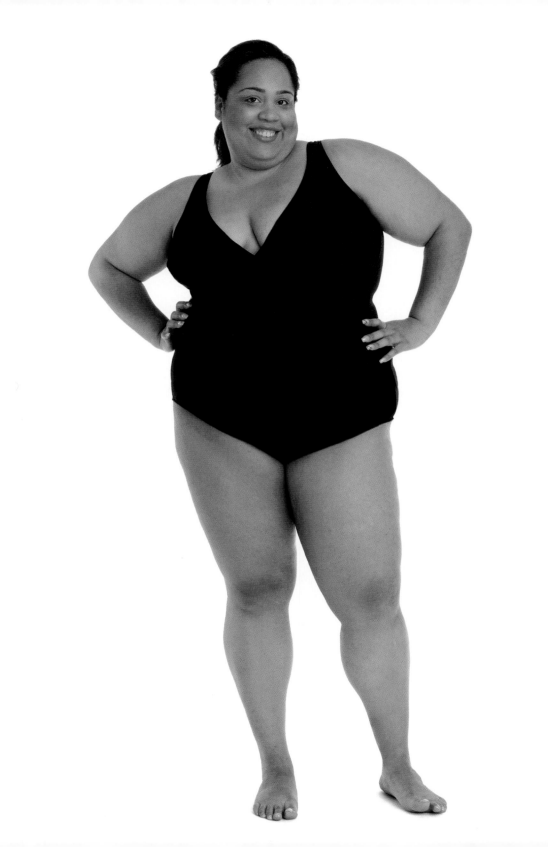

Extra Curvy,
Tall

EVELYN
5-foot-9
Size 28

"My biggest challenge is to find things that fall right on me. I'm constantly trying to find clothes that disguise my tummy. And I usually don't like wearing skirts because I feel like I have big thighs and skinny calves and ankles. I don't mind playing up my chest because these Girls look good in whatever I wear."

STACY AND CLINTON SAY: "Go, Evelyn! This is what we're going to help you do: bring lots more attention up toward your beautiful face and smile, play up your chest a little—not too much because we like to keep it tasteful—and use the narrowness of your lower legs while camouflaging the thigh."

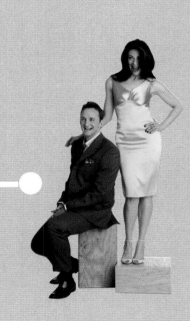

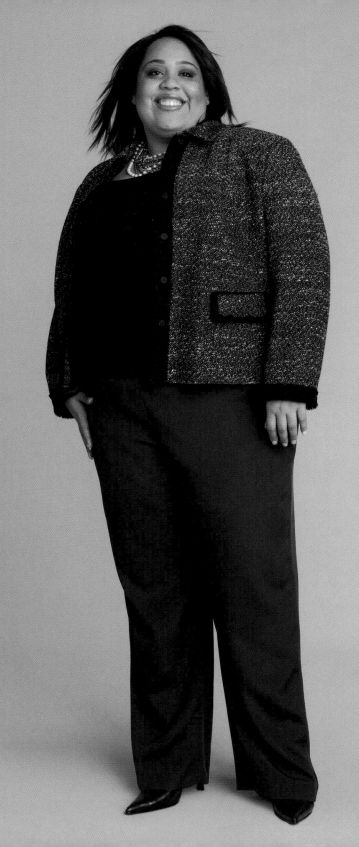

Extra Curvy,
Tall
Work

A jacket like this can work well to accommodate a heavier midsection as long as it is still fitted to the body line. A boxy tweed jacket is eternally classic. Mix it with pearls and it's eternally Coco Chanel classic.

Not only does this jacket help to camouflage a tummy, it actually helps to indicate a longer leg line by hitting at the top of the hip.

Deemphasize a larger torso with a darker top and a slightly lighter tone in the trouser.

Always go for a flat-front trouser! Plus-size designers make a lot of pleated pants, which simply does nothing to flatter the figure. You may have to look a bit harder to find a flat front and even go up a size or two to wear them correctly, but we promise, it's worth it for a longer, sleeker body shape.

Pointy-toe shoes elongate the leg with this midwidth trouser. (We know. We know. We keep saying it, so just wear them already!)

If you are going to do jewelry, keep it substantial. The multi-strand necklace is in proportion with Evelyn's frame and is strong enough to stand alone without other accessories. You could try an even longer multi-strand necklace as long as it doesn't hit any lower than the lowest button on the jacket.

Important Info About Jackets

Never ever buy a jacket you cannot close! We see women of all sizes do this, but it is a particular problem for plus-size women. The jacket fits you well in the shoulder, so it makes the body frame appear smaller. But it doesn't fit your midsection, so wearing it open becomes the only option. While we have no issue with you wearing your jacket open, we do when it's only because you can't close it. Wearing clothes that are too small will make you appear larger. Here are some tips:

1. *Always* buy jackets that fit the *largest* part of you, and have the shoulders taken in by a *tailor*. While not an inexpensive alteration, it is completely worthwhile and will make your jackets look more expensive and impressive.

2. Search for jackets with higher armholes. They fit more closely to the torso, clearly differentiating between the arm and the torso, creating a narrower silhouette.

3. Look for jackets with narrower arms. Wide sleeves can create bulk on the torso. If the body of the jacket fits well, then just have the arms taken in to create a sleeker silhouette.

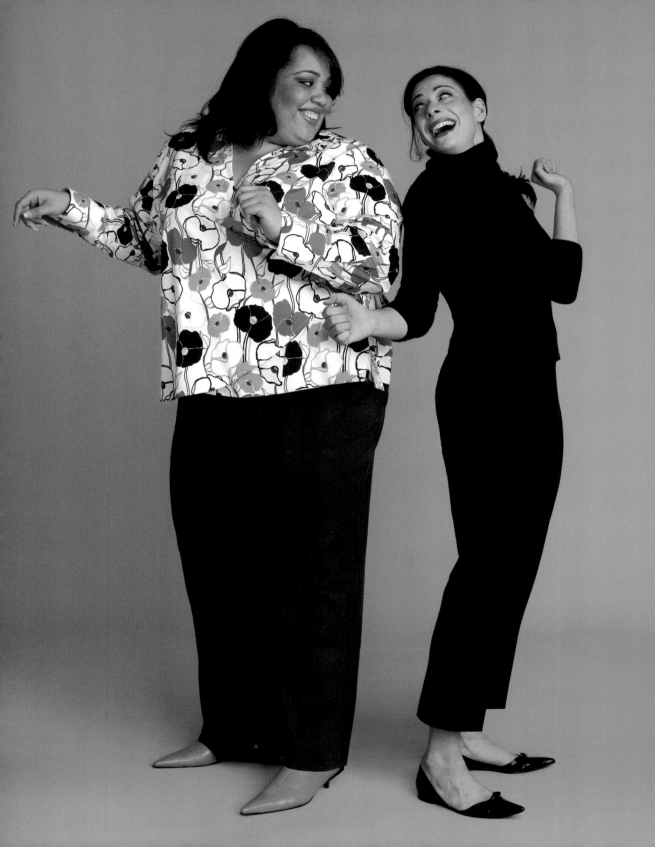

Extra Curvy,
Tall
Weekend

Choose prints that match the stature of your body. Too small a **print** would look childish on a larger frame.

A loosely fitting wrap shirt is an easy way to deemphasize a tummy and show some cleavage to feel sexy.

When you are a plus size, the wide-leg trouser in a midweight fabric is a true wardrobe staple. When you find a style that works well on you, buy multiples in a range of darker neutral colors.

Want a great coat option? Instead of dark brown, which might make this whole outfit look like a chocolate bar with flowers, try a lighter neutral in the brown family. A camel-colored coat would look great here.

Don't know how to incorporate print *and* color into an outfit? Choose a garment with great multicolor print and use the palette as your guide to add color accessories. Here, with a brown boot, try a pink bag. Or go for the opposite: pink heels and a brown bag. Your accessories don't have to match each other; they just have to "go." The outfit will still look cohesive because the print will bind together all of the colors in the outfit. Voilà!

Universal Tip: Beware of big accessories when wearing big prints. The print is the focus here. Don't add too much on top of it.

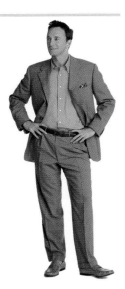

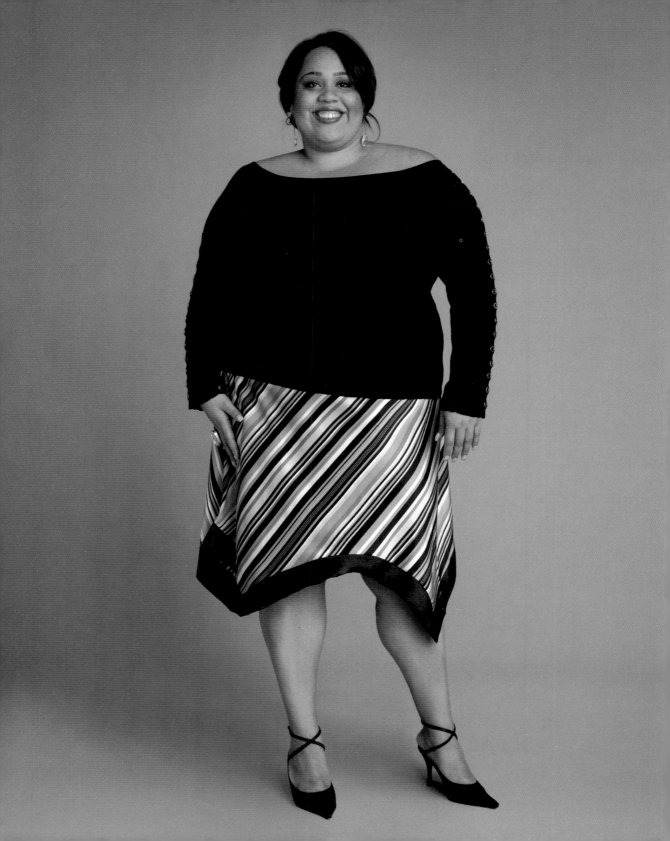

Extra Curvy,
Tall
Evening

A wider neckline on a sweater like this one adds drama to an evening outfit and keeps the attention up by the face.

The handkerchief hem is flirty and flattering to the legs, which don't appear as disproportionately skinny as Evelyn was afraid they might. If the skirt was longer, all we'd see is narrow ankle, throwing the body line out of proportion.

The diagonal variegated stripe on the skirt balances a wider torso and draws focus away from the top half and onto some seriously shapely legs.

With Evelyn's height she can easily wear a pointy-toe shoe with an ankle strap without breaking the line of the leg too severely. In fact, the ankle strap adds some definition to the ankle and keeps it in proprotion with the rest of Evelyn's frame, while echoing the stripe on the skirt to create cohesion in the outfit.

Add big jewelry to focal points for maximum impact: dangling earrings next to a bare neck or a big cocktail ring on a manicured hand. Very Lovey Howell from *Gilligan's Island*.

Hosiery Options: Evelyn could do a black sheer stocking here, but hose with back seams would look complicated with an ankle strap.

A vision of loveliness!

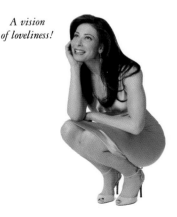

The Men

Essentials for Every Man

- A two- or three-button suit in a neutral color like black, charcoal gray, or navy in a heavier-weight wool
- A two- or three-button suit in a neutral color like brown or medium gray in tropical-weight wool
- A tweed sport coat
- At least six dress shirts (sized to neck and sleeve measurements) in a variety of colors
- Six sports shirts, long or short sleeve, like polos
- Six ties
- Two pocket squares
- Three sweaters, preferably cashmere
- An overcoat
- Brown loafers

- Black loafers
- Brown lace ups
- Black lace ups
- Two pairs of jeans: one in a medium wash for weekend, one dark for evening
- One pair of cargo, painter, or carpenter pants
- A brown belt
- A black belt
- A leather briefcase
- A quality umbrella
- A metal-banded watch
- A leather-strapped watch
- A nonathletic sneaker

(We're talkin' minimum here. Once you have these essentials, feel free to add like mad.)

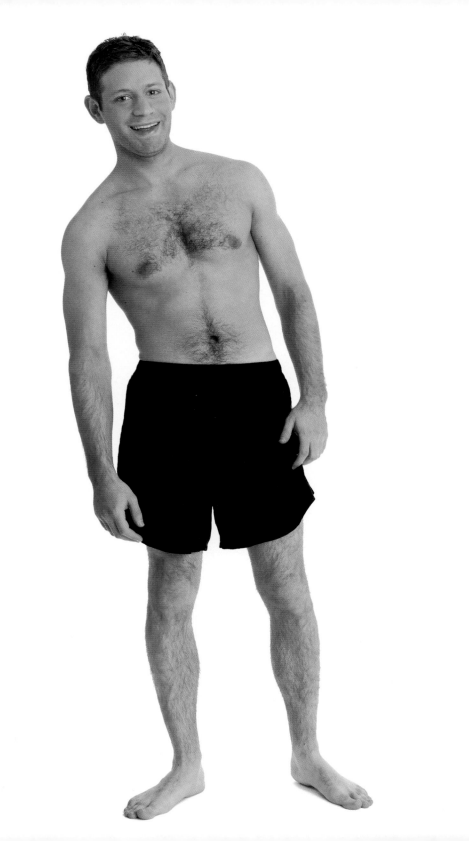

Short

DAN
5-foot-6
Jacket: 38
Waist: 32

"Short? Who says I'm short? I think I'm somewhere between short and average. I mean, I've seen guys shorter than I am, but, yes, most guys are taller. I think my rugged masculinity makes up for my, ahem, smaller stature, however. Do we have to talk about this? I'm still a little upset about not being allowed to ride a roller coaster until I was 18."

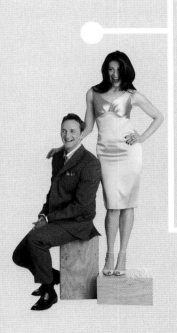

STACY AND CLINTON SAY: "Okay, Dan, let's get one thing straight: if you're short, you're short. This does not make you any less of a person. Just think of yourself as one hundred percent man with seventy-five percent of the packaging. (Okay, we're totally laughing right now as we write this because Dan is a friend of ours and we love giving him a hard time.) If you're short, there are a few pretty simple ways to make your body appear longer, the most significant of which is by creating the straightest, most streamlined silhouette possible. To do this, we eliminate excess fabric and pay close attention to the way clothes fit."

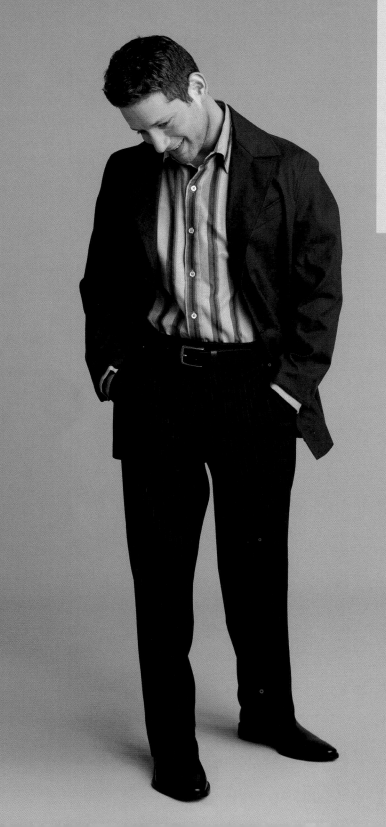

Short

Work

Shirts with strong vertical **striping** are an obvious yet nonetheless important way to add a little visual length—and therefore height—to a shorter-than-average frame. Tucking in not only looks neater but prevents you from looking like you're an eight-year-old wearing one of Dad's button-front shirts for art class.

Every man should own a classic trench—except perhaps you. A very long overcoat will only overwhelm your frame and make your legs look shorter. It's better for you to have a little distance between the hem of your coat and the floor, so get a topper coat like this one instead. Just make sure it's long enough to cover a suit jacket should you need it to.

When your tailor asks if you'd like a cuff on your pants, politely decline, then roll your eyes as if to say, "Duh." A cuff would only cut the line of the leg, and what we're going for here are longer lines. But note this: you'll have to look for flat-front trousers because pleated pants require a cuff.

Also keep an eye on that tailor of yours when it comes to the length of your trousers. You want your pants to have only a slight break (or fold) when they rest atop your shoe. Too much pooling of material at the hem of the trouser will only make you look shorter, and people may wonder whether you stole your pants from Grandpa.

Do a monochromatic belt, pant, and shoe combination for the longest line possible on the leg.

Universal Tip: When mixing stripes, let one be the focus (like the shirt here) and let another (like the pinstripe pants) play a supporting role to prevent clashing like a couple of divas on a stage.

To belt or not to belt your jeans?
There's certainly no rule about this, except that if you are going to do it, make sure the belt's a casual one. Any belt you'd wear with one of your best suits isn't one that should ever meet your denim, and vice versa. With denim, stick with cloth or flat leather instead of a polished leather.

Short
Weekend

A shorter, boxier jacket helps keep the torso wide and the legs long. The strong vertical stripe on the jacket also creates the illusion of length.

Because shorter men tend to have shorter necks, you're better off with shirts that have a low, or no, collar, like the kind found on a polo. Its soft collar lies flat and closer to the shoulder, creating a longer neck line. A V-neck tee would work just as well for this effect.

If you have a tough time finding shirts that don't seem to have been cut for a basketball player (because many of them do), you can have a tailor shorten the shirt so that the hem rests just an inch or two below that waistband of your pants. A less-expensive fix is to tuck in your shirt. Leaving it untucked and long just serves to shorten you by creating the illusion of shorter legs.

Once again, a dark shoe keeps the line of the leg intact. Avoid white or light shoes with **jeans** (à la Jerry Seinfeld in the late '80s); they will just break that **leg** line right up.

Universal Tip: If you're short and we see you walking around town with cuffed jeans, we're gonna come whop you upside the head. Cuffs shorten the leg's appearance—especially when they're a contrasting color.

Universal Tip: When choosing jeans, don't worry excessively about their length. More important, make sure you like the fit on the thigh and tush. Jeans can be expertly hemmed with their original stitching intact. Just request this from your tailor. If he's not catching your drift, tell him to use the same color thread as found elsewhere on the jean (usually gold) and to distress the new hem lightly with a little sandpaper.

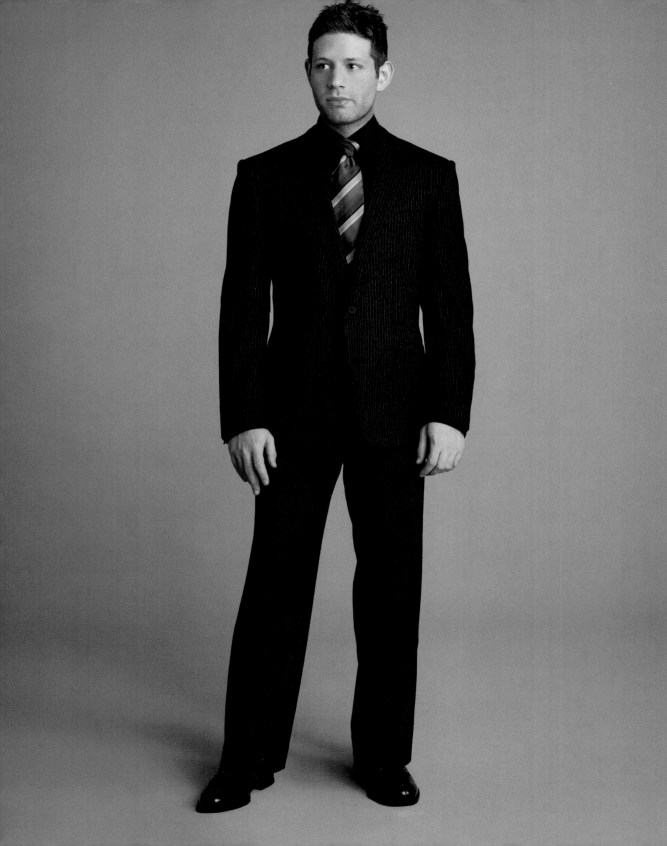

Short
Evening

You must not be embarrassed to walk into a store and ask for a *short* suit. Why not just get a regular if that makes you feel better? Because the goal is to create as streamlined an effect as possible, and the best way to do this is through the fit of your clothes. So get a jacket that ends where the tush meets the leg and have it tailored as closely to the body as is comfortable. A slight taper at the waist raises the visual center of the body to make the leg look longer.

Choose a two-button jacket with a moderately low stance. A lowish stance creates a long V on the torso and shows more of the tie. It helps your upper body appear longer.

Subtle pinstripes trick the eye a little; they're elongating but not overpowering to a smaller body.

Staying relatively monochromatic can also help you appear longer. The dark color of the shirt does not break the eye line at the neck and cuff, and, therefore, helps to create the streamlined look we've mentioned.

Note again the cuffless **pants** and the slight break at the hem.

Universal Tip: When trying on pants, be sure to consider your crotch. (Yes, we're talking about the crotch of your trousers, perv.) Don't allow the pants crotch to hang too far below your, uh, anatomical crotch. Not only will your body look out of proportion, your legs will appear shorter. If necessary, ask your tailor to take up the crotch in the rise a little. This may cause for an awkward measuring moment, but just go with the flow. And if you have to cough, remember to turn your head.

Seasonal Alternative: A black (or even dark gray) suit can seem out of place in the middle of the summer, except perhaps at a very fancy evening event. But this look would be just as snappy in navy, with the shirt and tie in any combination of blues.

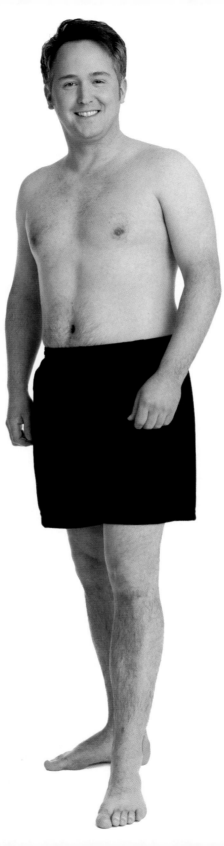

Average

JOHN
5-foot-10
Jacket: 40
Waist: 34

"I've always had what I guess is a pretty average body. I'm not too tall or too short or too big around the mid-section. So, I guess I'm pretty lucky when it comes to dressing, in that I don't have to think about it too much. I kind of just get up and go. I wouldn't mind, however, learning some of those finishing touches to help my style go from good to great."

STACY AND CLINTON SAY: "Okay, John, you asked for it, you got it. Because you do have a fairly easy body to dress, you will be our Everyman on whom we show how some beautiful classic pieces should fit."

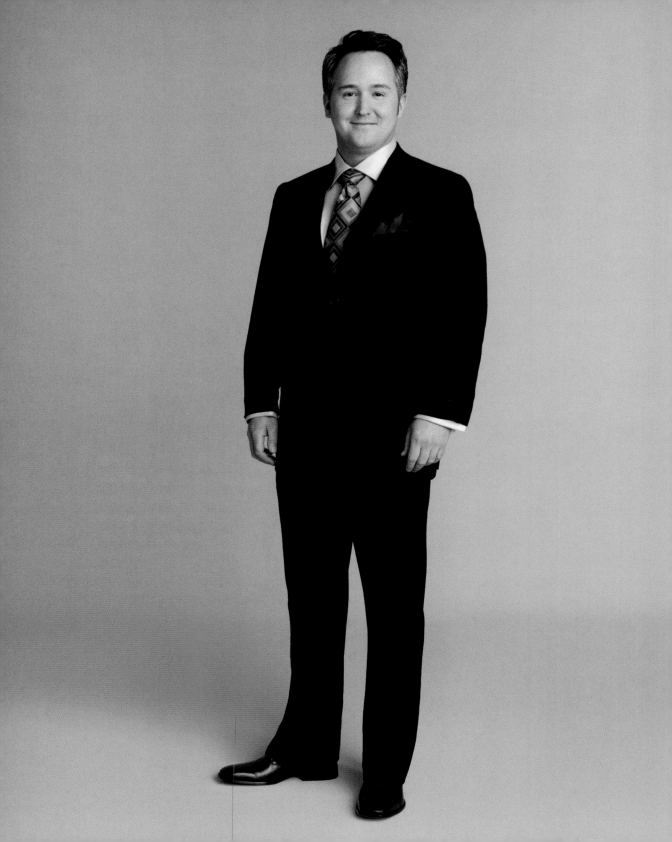

Average
Work

The two-button **pinstripe** suit is always a classic choice for the average-sized man, but without proper fit, he'll look just average. The first place to look for proper fit is the shoulder. You want to make sure the shoulder of the suit does not extend past your own natural shoulder but that you have a full range of motion throughout the shoulder when the jacket is buttoned.

Most men wear their suit sleeves too long. The sleeve of your jacket should cover your wrist, not your hand. And about a half-inch of shirt sleeve should show beneath that.

Don't be afraid to wear brown shoes with navy. It's a chic alternative to black. Some people say, however, that brown shoes aren't acceptable evening attire, which may be the case if you're attending a fancy event. But if you're going straight from work to dinner, they're completely proper, especially if they're dark brown—and well polished.

To cuff or not to cuff one's trousers is entirely up to the individual, but flat-front pants generally do not require one. Pants with pleats, however, do require cuffing to create a little extra weight at the bottom of the trouser in order to keep the crease sharp. And as we always say, too many pleats create excess bulk in the hip area—never a good look for a man. So, keep to a single pleat if possible.

Wear ties only with dress shirts, not sports shirts. Dress shirts are sized to one's neck and arm measurements. Sports shirts are sized S, M, L, and XL and are generally meant to be worn unbuttoned without a tie. You want to make sure you can fit two fingers into your buttoned collar for comfort and proper fit.

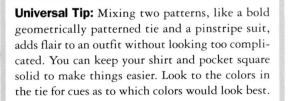

Universal Tip: Mixing two patterns, like a bold geometrically patterned tie and a pinstripe suit, adds flair to an outfit without looking too complicated. You can keep your shirt and pocket square solid to make things easier. Look to the colors in the tie for cues as to which colors would look best.

Every man should own a high-quality umbrella. Nothing cheapens a look more than the three-dollar number you bought outside a train station during a downpour.

Average
Weekend

The classic sport coat is wholly underutilized by the American man. It's the perfect way to look put together yet effortless. Think of it as the alternative to the sweatshirt or track jacket.

Once again, fit in the shoulder is essential. Just make sure the jacket is roomy enough so that you have full range of motion across the back and chest when buttoned.

Because you won't always wear your jacket with a long-sleeve button-front shirt, the jacket sleeves can be worn a little longer than those on your suit jacket. This will allow you to wear the jacket over even a short-sleeve T-shirt without feeling as though you're a teenager experiencing a growth spurt.

To keep your look young and modern, pair the sport coat with cargos, carpenter pants, or flat-front khakis. Such casual pants can be hemmed a little longer than dress pants for an intentionally slouchy, modern look.

Universal Tip: When mixing neutrals, like shades of brown and gray, add a pop of color somewhere in the outfit, like a sweater, to keep from looking lifeless.

Seasonal Alternative: Nothing says "fall" like a brown tweed sport coat, which is fine, except if it's June. So, for warm months, you might want to consider a linen jacket. But, please, buy a jacket that's a linen *blend*. One hundred percent linen wrinkles more than a shar-pei in a long hot bath. Granted, people expect linen to wrinkle and so they're more accepting of its creases, but the overall image can still be a sloppy one. Look for blends with cotton, silk, or synthetics for less mess.

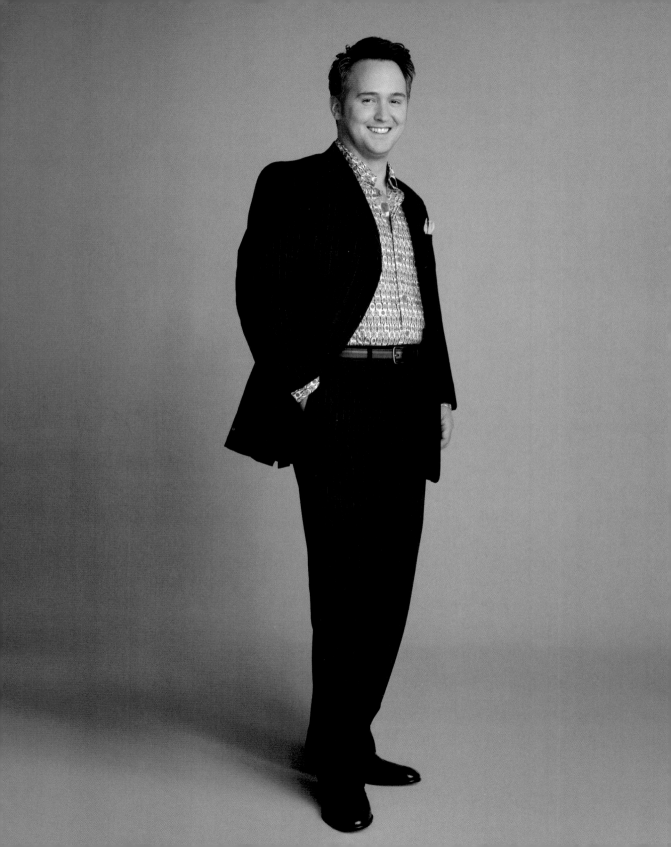

Average
Evening

The idealized man's body has a broad shoulder and a narrow waist. Suits with a strong shoulder construction help create this shape. You don't want so much padding that you look like Vanilla Ice in the '80s, but just enough to make your shoulder look broad, without the padding itself noticeable.

To help make your waist look smaller, ask your tailor to take the jacket in as much through the torso as possible without ruining the line of the suit.

If you're doing evening in a situation where a tie is not required, add interest to your outfit somehow, whether it's with a patterned shirt or pocket square or both. A solid open-necked shirt with a suit can look fine but dull. Why let women get all the attention at a party?

Make sure the color of your belt matches that of your **shoes**. (That should be obvious, but for some guys it's not.)

Universal Tip: Match your socks to your trousers, not your shoe. Except when you're wearing jeans. Then you can match the sock to the shoe.

Square Deal: For a pocket square that's dapper yet casual in feel, try a three-pointed fold. Just gather three points of the square in one hand and fold the last one back and under. Stuff it in your breast pocket so that the three points are visible. Don't show too much; you want to be stylish, not clownish. And either take the tag off the pocket square or make sure it's not visible.

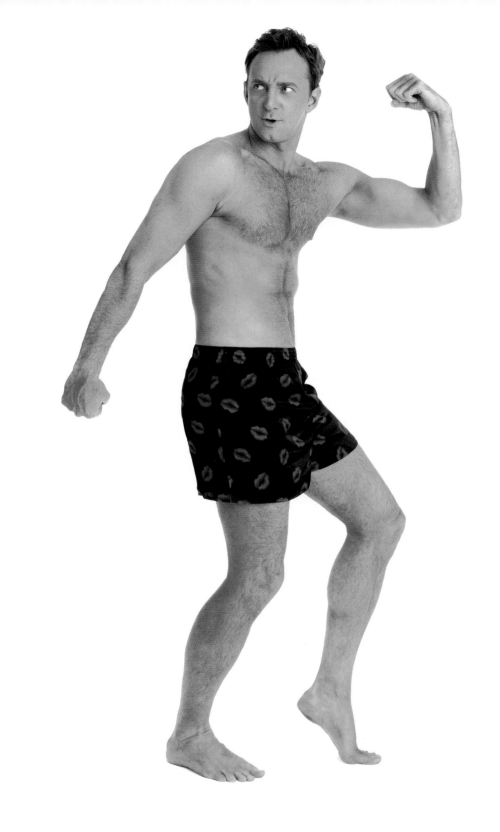

Tall

CLINTON
6-foot-4
Jacket: 42
Waist: 33

"I would say that at least half of the people who've seen me on television, then meet me in person say, 'I had no idea you were so tall!' And I never know how to respond. 'Ummm . . . thanks?' I've heard TV makes you gain ten pounds, but I didn't know it made you lose inches! In truth, there's a little part of me that wishes I could shave off four inches to be an even six feet tall, because that seems to be the cutoff point for most designers. I can't tell you how many shirts I try on that are just a little bit too short in the sleeve. It drives me nuts. But I also love being tall, especially when I'm dressed to the nines, because when you walk into a room, everyone notices. It's always a struggle, however, not to look gangly. Even though I have a medium frame, being tall makes you appear skinnier. So, following are tricks for tall guys who want to avoid looking like a newborn giraffe."

Please don't make me get naked again!

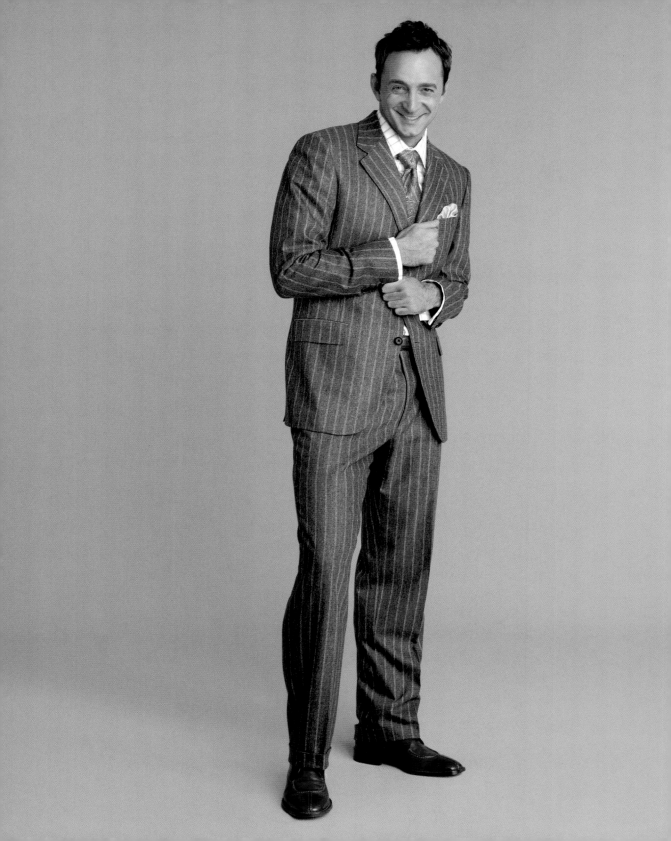

Tall

Work

A bold chalk stripe such as this one really plays up taller-than-average height and tends to work best on men with more body mass. Smaller-framed men will find this print a bit overpowering as opposed to a pinstripe.

A three-button suit with a slightly higher stance works well on tall men because it covers the surface of the torso and gives a less lanky appearance to the overall body frame. (We know, you can't see all three. But trust us, they're there.)

Just because you're tall doesn't automatically mean you need a "tall" suit. You may, but it's not a guarantee. If you're taller than 6-foot-4 you probably will. But if you're that height or shorter, try on the regular first. If the jacket is long enough to cover your butt, the length is fine. However, the length of the sleeve may need to be let out. Just make sure there is enough material to lengthen the sleeve accordingly.

If your trousers have a single pleat, they must have a cuff to weigh down the bottom of the trouser and keep the crease intact. And if they have more than one pleat? Leave them in the store. Seriously. There's really no need for more than one pleat. Added volume in the hip only makes you look, well, hippy. Not the ideal male silhouette.

Universal Tip: Instead of the obvious black shoe and belt with a gray suit, try brown for an elegant daytime look.

Seasonal Alternative: As beautiful as this suit is, it's definitely best when the temps drop—it's heavyweight wool-silk-and-cashmere flannel. A more versatile material is tropical-weight wool, a lighterweight fabric that allows for more air circulation, which should get you through three seasons: summer, spring, and fall.

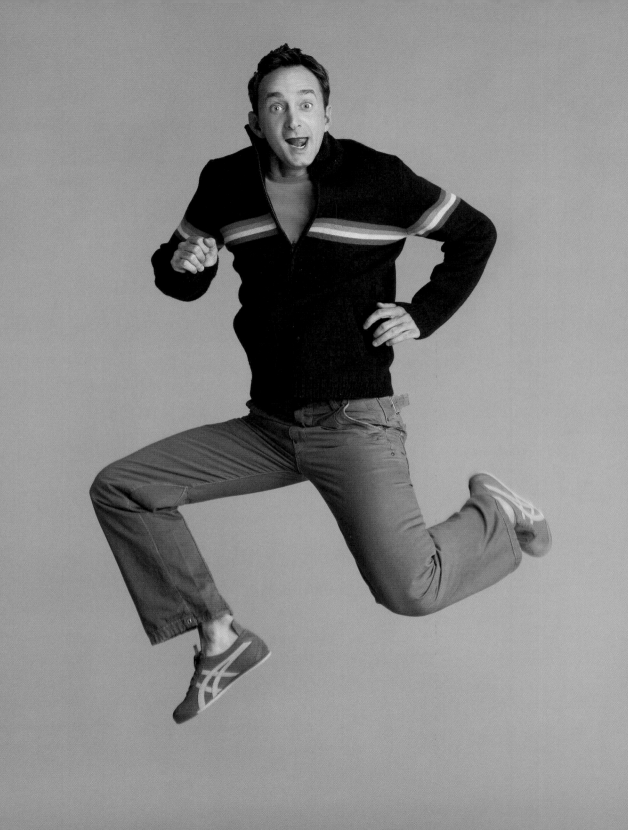

Tall
Weekend

Not every tall man has a long neck and face, but if you do (like Clinton), a stand-up collar on a sweater can deemphasize a narrow neck and facial structure. Along the same lines, a crewneck tee works better than a V-neck one, as the V just elongates the neck even more.

To give the impression of a broader chest and shoulder, look for tops with horizontal striping that extends across the chest and sleeve.

To keep from looking like a toothpick, choose pants that have a nice midwidth on the leg. Don't go too baggy, however, as you don't want your legs to end up looking disproportionately wider than your top half.

A contrasting shoe or sneaker breaks up the line of the body and adds a little extra visual interest.

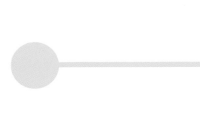

Universal Tip: There are three rules when it comes to going sockless and not looking like a schmo: (1) the shoe must be a casual one, like a sneaker or a soft loafer, (2) the occasion must be casual, like running to the grocery store or going on a picnic, and (3) the weather must be nice; you'll look dopey in a snowstorm without socks because that *is* dopey.

Shirt Tips: If you are tall but small- or medium-framed, you probably have a difficult time finding flattering off-the-rack button-front long-sleeve shirts that fit you perfectly. Either the sleeves will be too short or the torso too baggy. Basically, you have two options. (1) Find a shirt that fits the length of your arm, then have the torso professionally tailored to fit more closely in the midsection. (2) Choose a shirt that fits your torso well, then roll up your sleeves to mid-forearm; it's a look that's acceptable in casual offices and, of course, on the weekend.

Seasonal Alternative:
Obviously, you're not going to sport a turtleneck and velvet in the middle of August. But still, consider the idea of buying a jacket with a little extra sumthin' sumthin'—whether that's a bright contrasting pinstripe, a bold awning stripe, or even painted-on details. With the right fit, a special jacket makes a strong statement of style and confidence.

Tall
Evening

Tall men with average-sized frames have a tendency to look very narrow, so a printed jacket can add a little extra bulk to the upper body. It's also an excellent way to stand out a little for an evening in a sea of suits.

Turtlenecks work best on men with long necks or who have very broad shoulders. Be careful with the fit of your turtle, though. Too loose and it ends up looking feminine. Too tight and your **neck** ends up looking very skinny.

Velvet is a luxurious option for fall and winter. When mixing it, you need to do so with similar-weight fabrics, like denim, wool, or more velvet, like the pants shown here.

Your shoe should always be proportionate to your body. A tall man needs a long shoe to balance out his height, so if you have an average-sized foot on a tall body, look for shoes that have a slightly extended toe box. A note from Clinton: these are some crazy **shoes** I bought in Paris with a superextended toe box. I thought they were pretty bizarre, almost sci-fi. You don't have to go that extended, but I do think every man should own one pair of conversation-starting shoes.

Meow!

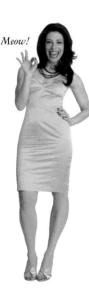

Universal Tip: To prevent the collar of your cashmere turtleneck from pilling, give yourself a nice close shave before going out for the evening. In fact, shave twice: once with the grain on the neck, then again against.

Universal Tip: There's a commonly held belief that you can't mix black with brown. Well, that's just freakin' wrong! While we don't advocate wearing a brown belt with black shoes, when it comes to clothing, not accessories, these neutrals work as well in combination as any others.

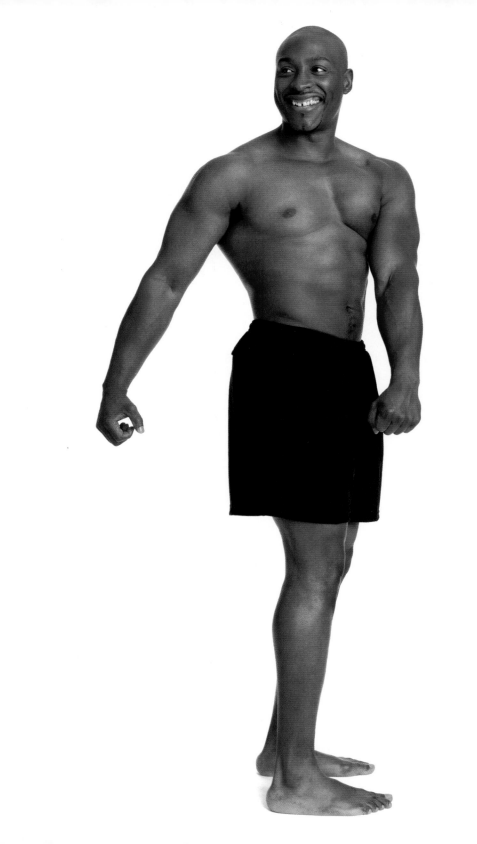

Athletic

MIKE
5-foot-10
Jacket: 44
Waist: 32

"I feel great about my body. I work out hard at least four times a week and watch just about everything I eat. If I had to pick a favorite part, I'd say my back. It's very broad at the top and tapers to a pretty narrow waist. My body does cause me a little hassle when I shop for clothes. Because I have big glutes, pants don't really sit right on me. If they fit in the butt, they're usually too big in the waist. And shirts can be a problem, too. If they fit in the shoulders, there's often a lot of extra material at the waist."

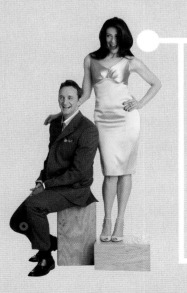

STACY AND CLINTON SAY: "Mike's body comes pretty darn close to that 'ideal' one we wrote about in the introduction: broad shoulders, narrow waist, the classic V shape. Ironically, even this body type poses its challenges because most clothes aren't cut with such a shape in mind. The average American man has more in the middle, and the average European isn't this broad in the shoulder. So, the athletic man can end up with a lot of extra fabric around the midsection or not fitting at all into some fashionable cuts. The trick is to use fabrics that cling to the body and find yourself a good tailor."

Universal Tip: Did you know that when you buy a belt, you should add two inches to your waist size? Yep. If you've got a thirty-two-inch waist, buy a thirty-four-inch belt; you won't look like you're hangin' on for dear life, and it'll give you enough room for an extra piece of Grandma's pumpkin pie next Thanksgiving.

Athletic
Work

If you've already got broad shoulders and high traps (those muscles on the sides of the neck), you have to be careful with jackets that have padded shoulders as you'll end up losing your neck and looking uncomfortable. That's why the softly constructed jacket is ideal for you. Softly constructed means that there is no padding added to the shoulder of the garment, so it lies flat against your natural shoulder. It's a style that can make narrow frames look even narrower, but here it works beautifully.

A multicolored, striped button-front shirt adds a little more verticality to a frame that has a tendency to look bulky. Don't be afraid to take a button-front shirt that you love to the tailor and ask for it to be more fitted at the waist. It's a pretty easy alteration—they just take it in a little in the back—and trust us, you will love the results: that V-shaped torso all men want.

If you work out your glutes a lot, you may find that trousers don't fit you perfectly right off the rack. They'll either fit you on the waist and be too tight on the butt, or they'll fit the butt and be too loose on the waist. That's where a gentleman's best friend—the tailor—should step in. Buy trousers that fit comfortably around the tush and have them taken in at the waist. That might add $10 or $20 to the cost of the garment, but it's money very well spent.

Do Us a Favor: Push yourself *just a little* when it comes to patterned shirts. Many men look at a shirt on a hanger or in a package and immediately say, "That's too bright!" or "That's got too many colors in it." Next time you go shopping, find your comfort zone—maybe it's a striped shirt with only two colors—then look for shirts that are slightly more intense somehow, such as with *three* colors or *brighter* colors. Then go try them on! We bet you a nickel you'll like what you see. (It's okay, you really don't have to send us the nickel. You already bought the book.)

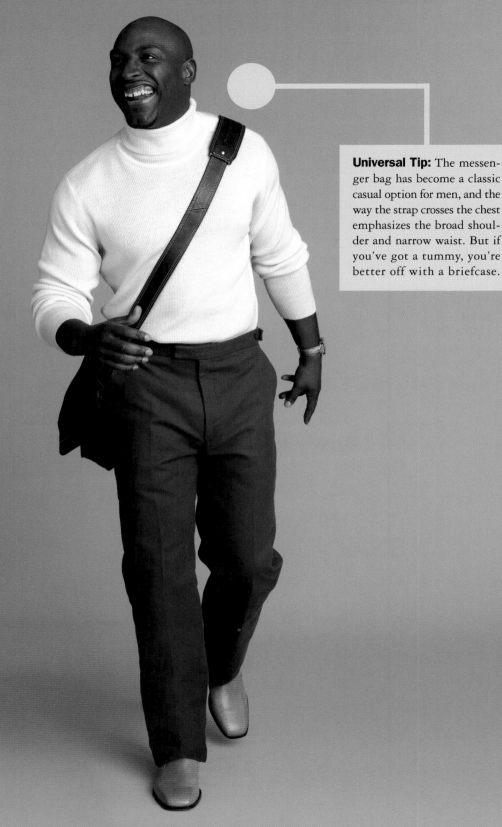

Universal Tip: The messenger bag has become a classic casual option for men, and the way the strap crosses the chest emphasizes the broad shoulder and narrow waist. But if you've got a tummy, you're better off with a briefcase.

Athletic
Weekend

Let's face it: when you've worked very hard to achieve a near-perfect body, you want to show it off, and nothing does that better than a clingy ribbed sweater. Plus, you won't have to worry about extra material at the waist or about armholes or shoulders that are too tight. Just make sure the rib is a fine one; you don't want to add any more bulk.

If Mike had a very thick neck, we'd suggest that he avoid turtlenecks. But he carries his bulk in his back and shoulders, so the turtleneck works nicely to balance those out. The color of the sweater also makes a big difference. Because there's a nice contrast between his skin tone and the sweater, we're not losing Mike.

When doing just two colors, especially neutrals, add in different **tones** in the accessories.

> **Universal Tip:** Some quick notes about matching accessories.
> • Does a belt have to match the shoes? Not exactly, but they should be roughly the same color. If Mike's pants had belt loops, he could wear a brown belt, not necessarily the same brown in the shoe.
> • Does a watch have to match anything? Not so much for daytime. Most leather-strapped watches are neutral anyway, so they can be worn with most everything else.
> • Does a bag have to match anything? Once again, no. While a man looks very put together when his accessories are all in the same color family, he doesn't necessarily look sloppy when they aren't.

Seasonal Alternative: Too hot for a cashmere turtleneck? Go for a lightweight cotton ribbed T-shirt in either a crew or V-neck. Same great fit, a lot less perspiration.

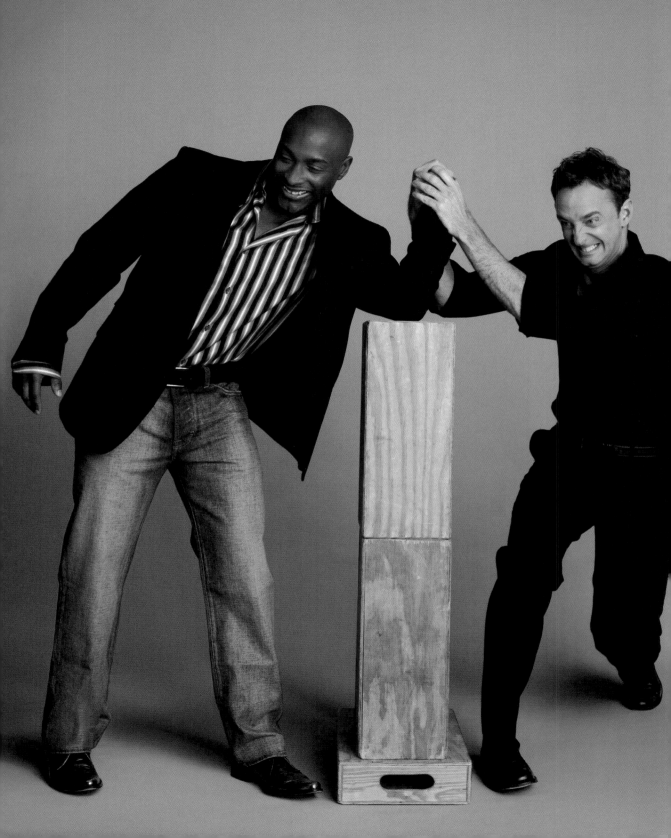

Athletic
Evening

The tuxedo jacket is a chic option for nighttime and creates a very streamlined look. The broad lapel plays up a strong shoulder line.

The striped shirt, once again, gives a little more vertical emphasis to a frame that could otherwise look too broad. Tucking it in shows off the naturally narrow waist.

The wide-leg jean will provide more comfort and the lighter wash makes the legs appear a little thicker, bringing balance to the overall look.

Here the sleeve of the jacket was left intentionally long for a very modern, casual evening look. Obviously, if Mike were attending a formal event and needed a full tux or suit, the sleeve should be shortened to not cover the hand. And here, we've unfolded the French-cuff shirt so that it sticks out beyond the sleeve of the jacket. It says, "Yes, I know my sleeve is long, and that's the way I want it. You only wish you could look this good."

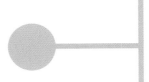

Universal Tip: Metallic shoes aren't just for women. Mike's pewter-colored ones add a little extra interest to the outfit. Don't bother trying to find a metallic belt to coordinate. That would look a little too matchy-matchy.

A Quick Word About "Athletic" Suits: This term is generally used to define a suit with a drop of more than seven inches. The traditional drop is six inches. To determine your drop, subtract the waist size from the jacket size; Mike's drop is twelve inches, which means that any suit off the rack will have to be altered considerably for a perfect fit. A forty-four jacket usually comes with a thirty-eight-inch waist, so in Mike's case, the pants would have to be taken in quite a bit. Suit separates may prove to be an easier option, and they're becoming more and more popular in department stores. That way, Mike could buy a forty-four jacket and a thirty-two trouser separately but in the same fabric.

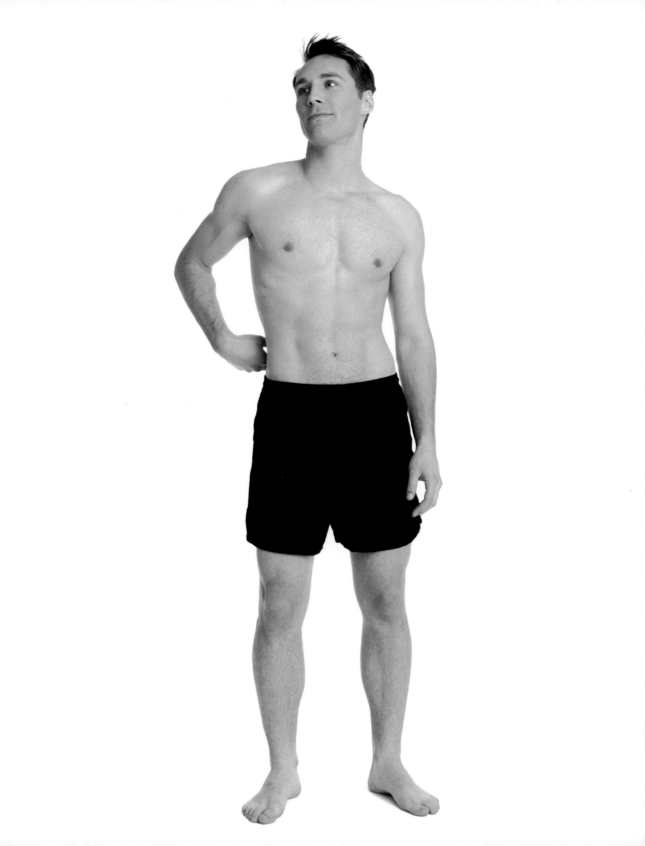

Small-Framed

JOSH
5-foot-10
Jacket: 36
Waist: 30

"My first response when you guys asked me if I'd be your representative for the 'small-framed man' was 'I'm not small-framed!' Maybe I'm in denial over it. No, I'm kidding, really. I know I'm small-framed, but I don't go around thinking of myself as skinny. I feel like most men's clothes are designed with a bigger man in mind, so it's difficult to find clothes that are proportioned right. But when I do find clothes that fit, I like the line of my body, very long and fluid and minimalistic."

STACY AND CLINTON SAY: "Josh definitely isn't the average Joe when it comes to his mind-set about his body. We've found through very scientific research (well, sort of) that if you ask 100 American men for their clothing size, 93.5 of them will reply, 'I'm a large.' We're not 100 percent sure why, but there's definitely some kind of American stigma attached to being anything smaller than a large. Josh, however, realizes that sometimes he's a medium and sometimes he's a small. And that's the key to best dressing the narrow frame."

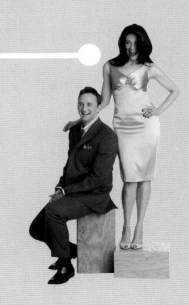

Wearing white by your face can make your teeth look yellow, especially if you have pale skin. Make sure those choppers sparkle, or go with an off-white or pastel.

Small-Framed
Work

When it comes to suiting, European designers (particularly the French and Italians) cut a lot narrower than American designers, because, quite frankly, the average American is a lot bigger than the average European. So, we recommend putting your patriotism aside and at least trying on an Italian or French suit if you've got a smaller frame. You'll see how much closer to your body they **fit**—and you won't feel, for a change, as though you've got enough room for you and a small family under your jacket. By the way, the Europeans cut their pants with a slimmer leg, too.

If you drive a Chevy and prefer a good old cuppa joe to a cappuccino, you *can* find American-made suits that work on a small frame. Just don't be afraid to ask your tailor to narrow the arms and torso so they look like you fill out the suit.

Keep the lapels on your jacket narrow, in proportion with the rest of the body. A huge lapel would only look clownish.

The same goes for your ties. Err on the side of narrower, no matter what the current trend.

If you've got a narrow face to go with your narrow bod, a spread collar can help balance out that skinny skull. (A spread collar, by the way, is one on which the points have a little distance between them. They sort of *spread* out over the shirt.) There's a catch, however: spread collars require tie knots large enough to fill that gap. *But,* if you're small framed, you don't want the size of your knot to be as big as your head. So . . . try the half-Windsor. Whaddya mean, you don't know how to tie one? Go look it up on the Internet right now, fella.

Universal Tip: It goes without saying (but we're gonna anyway) that you *never* button the bottom button on your suit jacket. When it comes to the top button, however, you can take into account your own personal taste and the construction of the lapel. If the lapel rounds softly over that top buttonhole, leave the button undone so as not to create any unsightly creases or pulling.

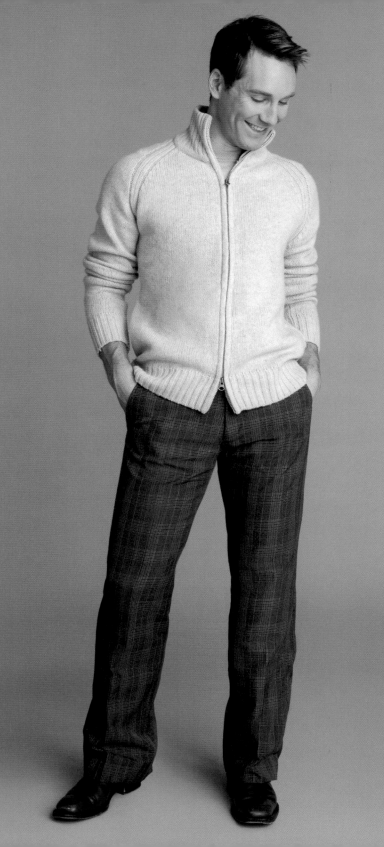

Small-Framed
Weekend

An easy way to make your upper body appear larger than your lower is to wear a lighter color on top and a darker color on the bottom.

Thicker knits can also add a little extra width to a small frame. Just don't do thick and oversized. You'll look like *you're* the one who shrank in the wash.

Look for details that add extra emphasis to the shoulder. This sweater has a raglan sleeve (note how the sleeve is one piece from the wrist to the collar), which has a tendency to make the shoulder appear larger and more defined. Baseball jerseys with contrasting-colored arms are another way to achieve this effect.

The last thing you want when you have a small frame is to look like a little boy who's playing dress-up in Grandpa's big, baggy pants. That only makes you look smaller. So look for slim fits in casual pants. Trust us, you'll look bigger if you fill out clothes with a slimmer construction.

Your attention to fit should extend all the way down to your T-shirts. Oversized tees will only make you look scrawny. Look for fitted tees in *small* sizes. You're not large, so don't buy anything with the L-word on the label.

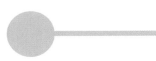

Universal Tip: Cream—it's an essential neutral but can be deadly on light skin, making you look washed out. It works best when there's even just a little color, like this light blue tee, up by the face.

Seasonal Alternative: A track jacket would be a nice substitute for this wool sweater when the weather gets warmer, especially when mixed with a dressier pant. Just be sure to buy one that fits close to the body. Another perfect look for a small-framed guy: a fitted short-sleeve tee worn *over* a fitted long-sleeve one.

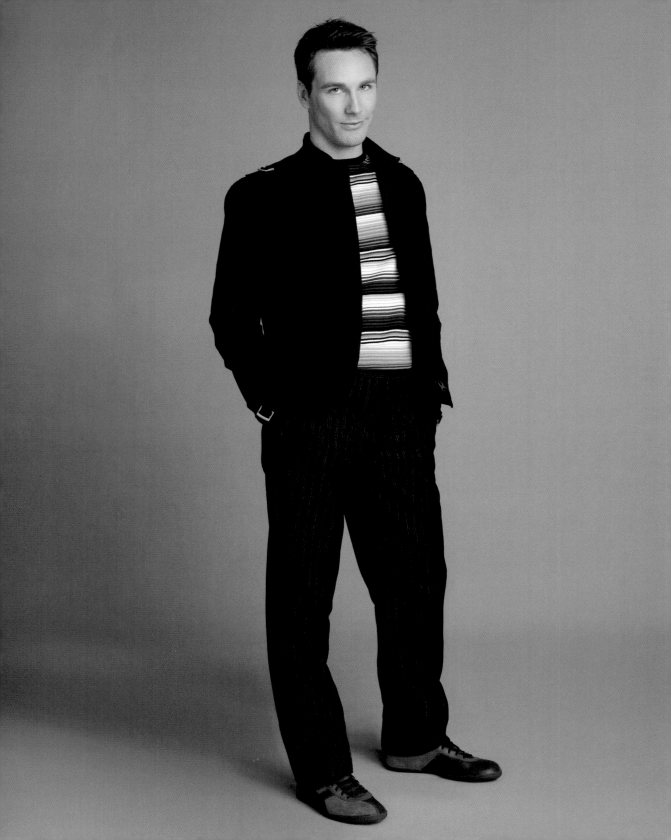

Small-Framed
Evening

We often say that horizontal stripes across the tummy only make the tummy appear larger. This is not the case, however, when your tummy is nonexistent. Here, the horizontal stripes in bold colors add a little width to the top half. The open jacket, though, keeps the line nice and lean.

Like the raglan sleeves in the previous example, epaulettes are another way to add shoulder emphasis.

A quick word on trends and how to follow them: military details—and epaulettes certainly fit into that category—go in and out of fashion on a very regular basis. Some seasons you'll hear, "It's all about military for fall!" and by the following spring military is "so over." To keep your wardrobe from losing its value overnight, invest in trends in moderation, spending only what you can afford to take as a loss should that look quickly go out of style. *Or,* look for pieces that subtly follow a trend. We'd consider this jacket a good investment because it doesn't *scream* military. If it were army green and covered in patches, that would be another story.

Also, you're better off with jackets, like this one, that have a boxier construction. Why? Because boxier = shorter on waist and wider on torso. That gives the appearance of a broader upper body and a narrow waist.

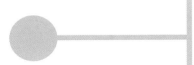

Universal Tip: You can do sneakers for evening if . . . they're not "athletic" sneakers *and* if their design is harmonious with the rest of your ensemble *and* if you're just hanging out with your friends. If these were muddy and covered in grass, they obviously wouldn't work. If they were orange, they wouldn't be so appropriate for a night out, but might be fine for day. And if Josh were heading to a wedding dressed like this, we'd slap him upside the head.

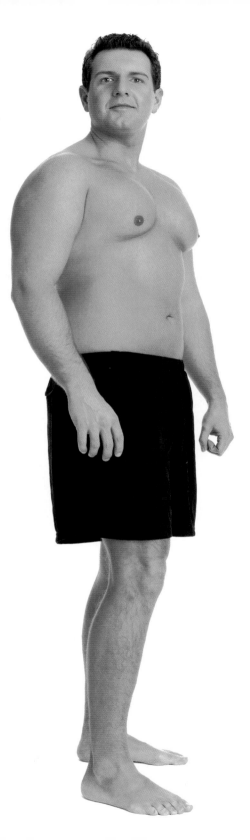

Barrel-Chested

MIKE
6-foot-2
Jacket: 44
Waist: 36

"I love my body. I love everything about it. I'll even go so far as to say I have the best body in this book—except maybe for that guy over there who looks like he works out twenty-four hours a day."

STACY AND CLINTON SAY: "Typical Mike (who's a good friend of ours) with a level of self-esteem that's off standardized psychological charts. We asked Mike to represent barrel-chested types like himself to show how men built like him can play up their large chest, arms, and shoulders without bringing too much attention to a thicker midsection. Not that you aren't perfect, Mike."

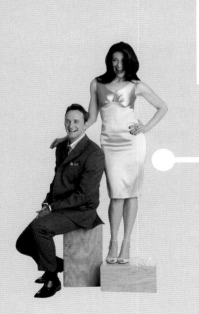

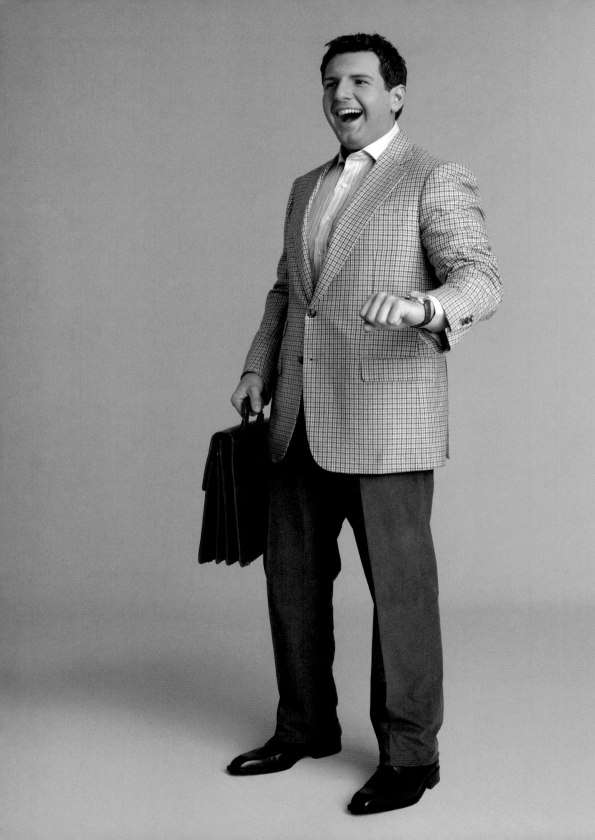

Barrel-Chested
Work

Big men can handle more **pattern** than smaller men, so to stand out, experiment with checks or houndstooth or glen plaids.

Doing a light color like this on top really plays up a strong chest and shoulder, but the line of the jacket camouflages any extra bulk in the midsection. Fit in the shoulder, as always, is extremely important here. If the jacket were too constricting, Mike would give off the impression that he's outgrowing his clothes. Not such a professional look. And if the jacket were too large, he'd look sloppy.

A big man needs a big **watch** for proportion. A slim one would look too dainty.

The flat-front fine-wale cords in brilliant blue are a bold choice, much more European in feel than American. Obviously, they're not necessary for dressing a barrel-chested body type, but they do serve to bring some attention to the lower half and their straight lines add a little more length to the leg.

Universal Tip: The idea of mixing stripes (the shirt) and plaid (the jacket) is enough to send the average guy running for solid ground. However, it's not all that difficult. First, find the common color. In this case, the light blue in the shirt picks up the light blue in the jacket. Second, vary the "weights" of the patterns. The shirt's pattern is a subtle one, whereas the jacket's is bolder. You can mix two subtle patterns, but two bold ones becomes a trickier mix. Pick a primary pattern and let the other play a supporting role.

Universal Tip: A leather-strapped watch integrates well for work or daytime. It's not essential that you match the color of the leather—in this case brown—to your belt, shoes, and briefcase, but it's nice when you do.

Universal Tip: When choosing sunglass frames, look for shapes that are the opposite of your face shape. For example, round frames only make round faces look rounder. But a squarish frame like the ones shown help balance a roundish face.

Barrel-Chested
Weekend

A V-neck sweater elongates the neck a little and prevents Mike from looking too bulky on top.

The long-sleeve T-shirt in a contrasting color underneath brings the eye up toward the face. The white sleeves showing at the wrists help to pull the outfit together and look more finished.

A boxy **sweater** provides extra room without clinging on the sides. Avoid ribbing on the bottom of a sweater; it will only emphasize what's above it. However, this sweater is ribbed on the arms and shoulder, so it clings to the parts you'll want to show off.

A big macho man like Mike needs a substantial lug-soled shoe to balance his large upper body.

Forest green and purple: one of our favorite color combinations.

Universal Tip: If you're barrel-chested and shorter than Mike, who's pretty tall at 6-foot-2, you might find that the sweaters that fit your shoulders and tummy hang down past your crotch. What's a guy to do? Tailor, tailor, tailor. Not all knits can be shortened, but most can. So, keep your receipt when you shop and head straight for the dry cleaner (or whoever else does your tailoring) on your way home from the mall. If the sleeves and hem can be taken up, keep it. If not, return for a full refund.

The Dreaded Catalog Sweater: With this body type, avoid at all costs what we call the "catalog sweater." You know it when you see it: man and woman sitting in a ski lodge by a roaring fire, sipping cognac, wearing chunky (usually red) sweaters with big snowflakes and/or reindeer. Not only is this the male equivalent of the snowman-appliqué holiday sweater worn by many a grandma, it's universally unflattering—especially for you. The last thing you need is a humongous, patterned, wool sweater adding bulk to your upper body.

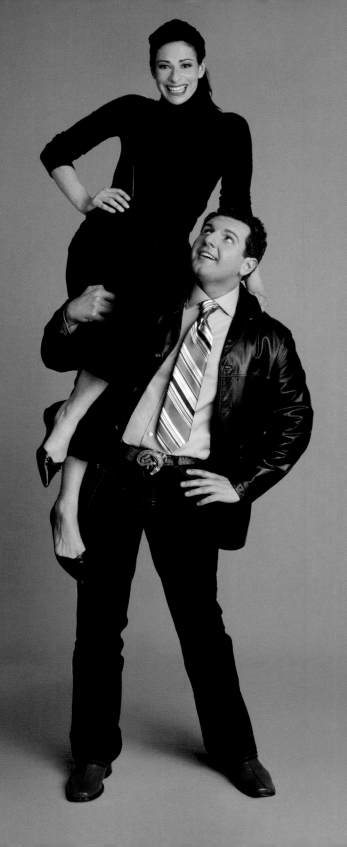

Tie One On

Don't think of ties for just formal affairs or work—and they don't always require a jacket. You can look very stylish wearing a beautiful tie with a crisp, well-fitting button-front shirt. When the jacket's off, roll your sleeves up, even to the elbow. Otherwise you might end up looking like you've left your jacket at the coat check.

Barrel-Chested
Evening

When you're very broad on top, it's essential that you add a little width to your lower half for balance or you'll end up looking like those guys at the gym who have no necks and toothpick legs. So a wide-leg jean is your best bet. Low-rise jeans can emphasize a tummy, so look for medium rise instead.

When you're tucking in your shirt, don't jam it in there so it's tight. Blouse it a little so it pulls away from the tummy.

A tie always helps create a strong vertical line. A wider one with a bold print is more appropriate for a larger guy.

The car coat is ideal for this body type. It's got a soft-shoulder construction, so it plays up naturally strong shoulders without adding any more bulk. And the long straight line is very elongating and camouflages any extra girth in the midsection.

A bold three-dimensional belt **buckle** looks at home on a barrel-chested man; on a smaller frame it would overwhelm.

Universal Tip: When tying your tie, aim for the top of your belt, especially when you want to show off the buckle. In general, shorter is chicer than longer.

Seasonal Alternative: Lightweight suede is always a nice option for spring and summer if the leather's not letting you breathe enough. See page 198, for an example of a softly constructed jacket that would easily work for you, too.

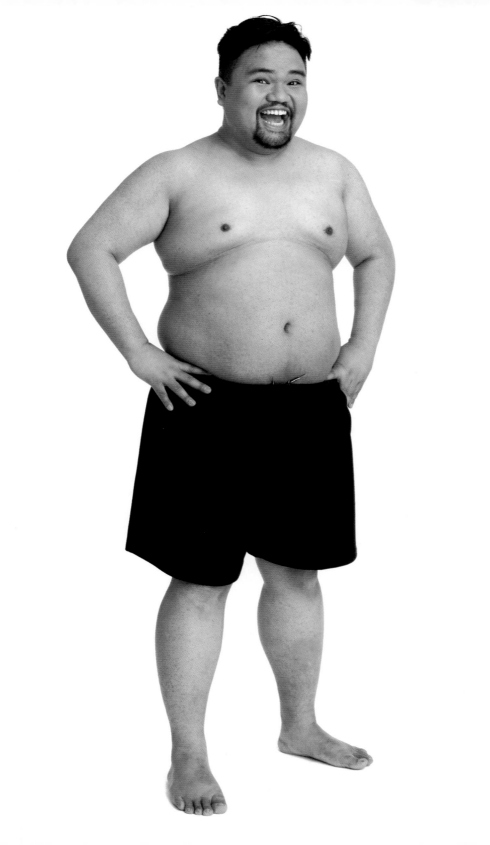

Tummy

OMAR
5-foot-9
Jacket: 40
Waist: 46

"Okay, I'll take my shirt off, but I'm not gonna like it."

STACY AND CLINTON SAY: "Thanks, Omar, for being a good sport. So, you've got a tummy. It's not like you're the only one. The key to dressing when you've got extra in the middle is to create balance throughout the rest of the body with stronger shoulders and wider legs. That way, the tummy won't seem out of proportion. You'll just seem big and strong all over!"

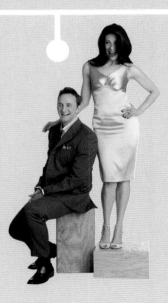

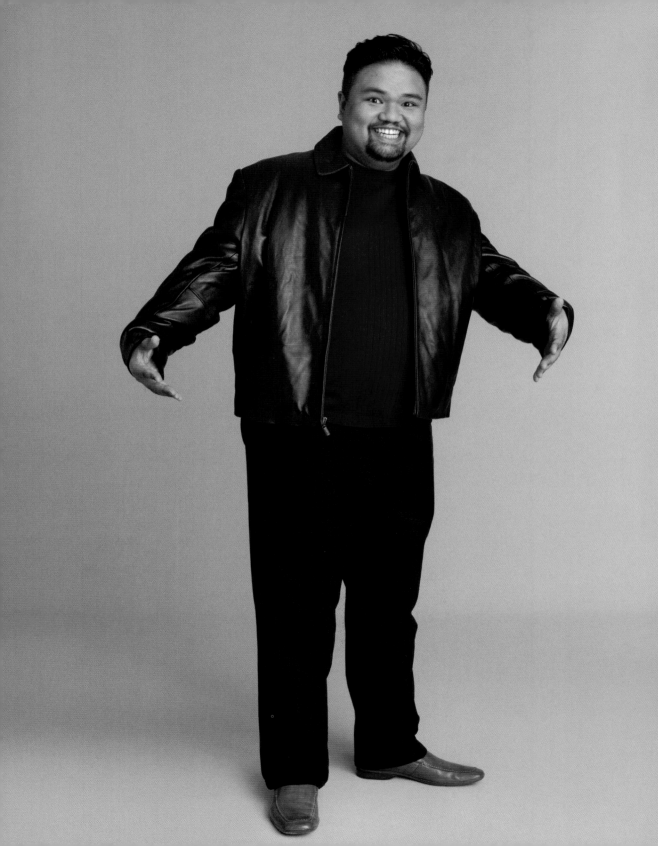

Tummy
Work

Boxy jackets work best on men with a little extra in the middle because they're roomier in the midsection, providing more comfort and lending the appearance that the jacket is what's creating bulk. A strong shoulder construction, meaning even a small shoulder pad, is also important here, as it balances out the larger tummy.

When it comes to jackets especially, stick to stiff fabrics, like leather, because they control your shape better than flimsy ones. Also, they just look more suitable to your frame.

Wide, straight-leg trousers are superimportant for the man with a tum-tum. So much menswear for the larger guy comes with tapered (narrower at the ankle) legs, we could pull out our hair. It's exactly the opposite of what you want to be doing. A narrow ankle only makes everything above it look wider in comparison. We call this the ice-cream cone effect. We don't know any man who's name isn't Häagen-Dazs who wants to be compared to a waffle cone. So buy the widest-leg trousers you can find and don't give up the fight!

When doing knitwear, avoid clingy cuts. A vertical rib, like the one on this sweater, helps create verticality rather than horizontality. And don't do a ribbed waistband; boxier is better. A waistband would only cling below the belly and emphasize it.

Pull your trousers up as high as possible on the tummy, especially when you're wearing an untucked sweater over them, because you don't want a saggy crotch. That only shortens the leg—and looks damn sloppy.

No pleats, no matter what. There are a lot of trousers out there with 'em, but keep on walking by. Multiple pleats only add bulk to the groin area. And we don't want that.

Seasonal Alternative: Too hot for leather? Go for a boxy denim jacket, the darker the wash the better, or corduroy, the ribs of which will also provide a subtle vertical line.

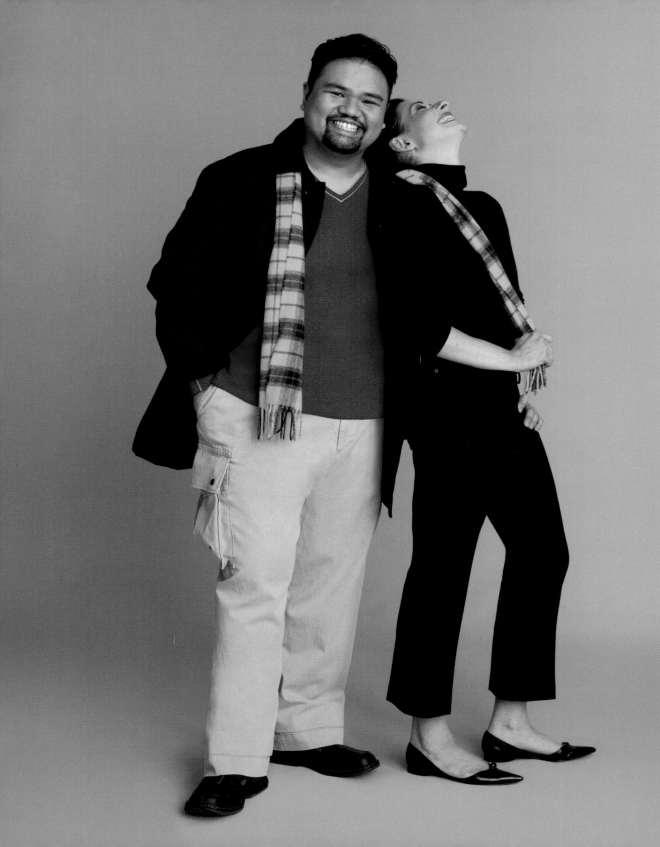

Tummy

Weekend

Car coats, topper coats, or pea coats (the kind longshoremen wear) are usually generously cut and create a long straight line from the shoulder to the top of the thigh, thereby tricking the eye away from the midsection.

A cargo pant with side pockets adds a little extra bulk to the lower body, which really works in Omar's case to balance his lower half with the upper. This is especially important for men with wider midsections and narrower limbs because it gives the impression of "big framed" rather than "beer gut."

The V-neck sweater helps elongate the neck a little, which always helps elongate the entire person.

Even an accessory like a scarf can do a lot to add vertical emphasis. Some guys are antiscarf, which kind of confounds us. They're very dapper and they keep your neck warm on a cold day. Plus, they're the best way to hide a hickey.

For casual looks, keep the shoe chunky. A big guy needs a nice big shoe to roam around town in. It's more in keeping with your body proportion. Ever see a skinny little guy in huge combat boots? Looks kinda silly, right? But you could pull that off if you wanted to.

Is it legal to look this hot?

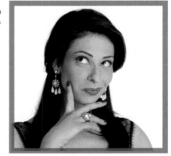

Seasonal Alternative: For warmer temps, try a boxy polo or a bowling-style shirt. They're cut with extra room in the midsection and can be worn untucked so as to deemphasize a tummy.

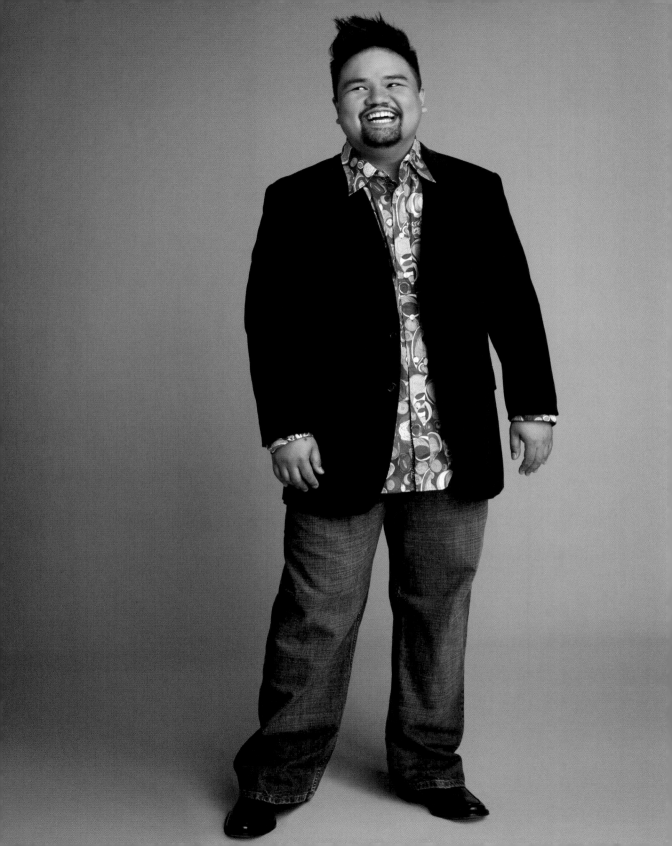

Tummy
Evening

See, black *is* slimming—when it fits well. The key here is that the jacket fits perfectly in the shoulder, and even though Omar's a big guy, we can still see the tailoring in the sides. The jacket cuts in at the waist.

The bold design of this button-front shirt is in keeping with Omar's stature (a dainty one would be too subtle) and the irregularity of the print is camouflaging. On the contrary, a stripe can be tricky if you've got a tummy. If the line bows out, it would accentuate the curve of the body.

Keep the **shirt** untucked to camouflage the tummy, but be careful with the length. Any lower than the bottom of the crotch and you might look like you're wearing a dress.

This look is obviously for casual evening, so leave the jacket open. Notice how it creates a nice long straight line down the front of the body, especially because of the sharp contrast between the bright pattern and the solid black jacket.

There's the perfect example of a wide-leg jean balancing the upper body.

We left these jeans intentionally long for extra volume on the leg. There's just a little bit of pooling to draw the eye downward. If the lines elsewhere weren't so strong, this would make Omar look shorter, but here it obviously doesn't.

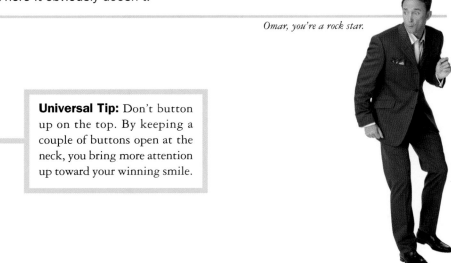

Omar, you're a rock star.

Universal Tip: Don't button up on the top. By keeping a couple of buttons open at the neck, you bring more attention up toward your winning smile.

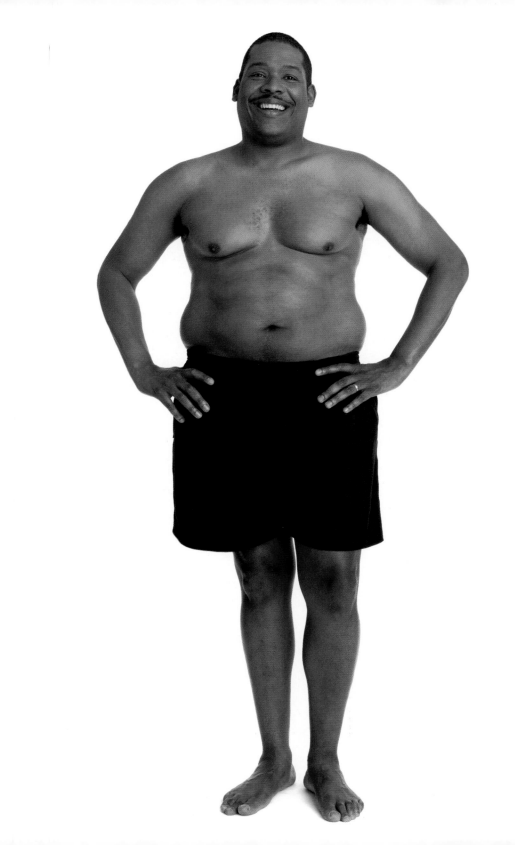

Hips

TONY
6-foot-3
Jacket: 44
Waist: 46

"I carry my weight pretty low on my torso—on my sides and my hips—which is pretty rare for a guy. Definitely frustrating because I feel like what's available in stores doesn't match my body."

STACY AND CLINTON SAY: "This body type is not as uncommon as you may think. We've actually dressed it many times. The key in dressing it best is balancing out the lower body by adding more emphasis to the upper."

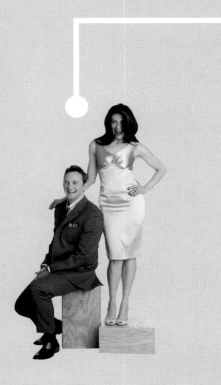

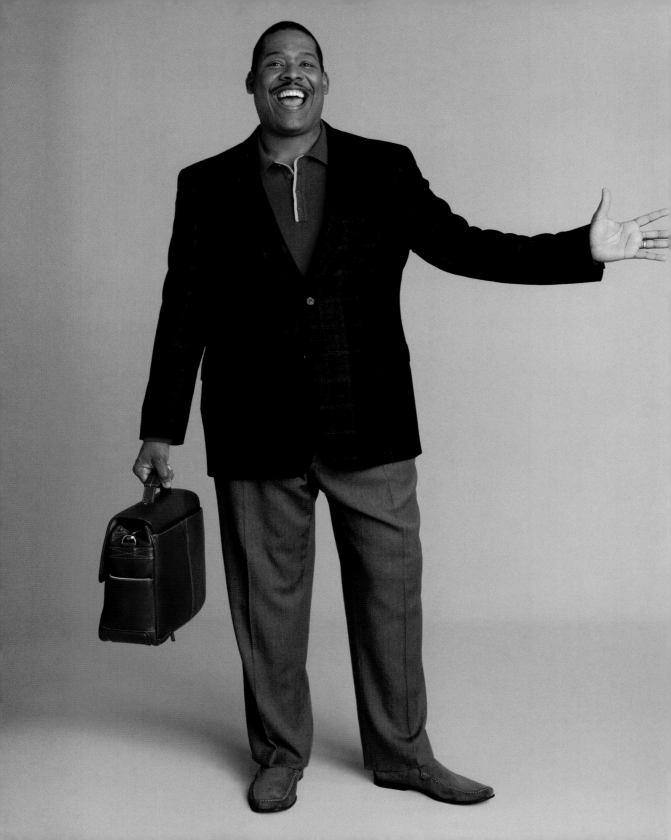

Hips
Work

If you carry the bulk of your weight on your lower half (hips and love handles), a sport coat can be your best friend in helping to camouflage it.

When it comes to jackets, American designers generally cut for a larger frame. In this case you would want to make sure the jacket is slightly boxy (yet tailored slightly through the middle) and long enough to cover the widest part of you. (Women take note: this rule of thumb does not apply to you.)

By putting a bright color under the darker-color jacket, we bring attention up to the face and away from any problem areas.

The bigger man you are (we're talking about your stature, not your character), the more pattern you can carry on your frame, like this windowpane. (The horizontal and vertical stripes intersect, forming a grid.) It makes the look a little more interesting than a plain navy blazer with tan trousers.

Keep accessories, like a briefcase, proportionate to body size. Tony would look pretty silly carrying around a little bag.

If you do carry your weight low on your body, that's probably the best excuse to wear pleated pants, because you need a little extra room. But stay with a single pleat if you can. It just looks neater.

Universal Tip: We get asked a lot, "When should I put my shirt collar outside the jacket?" The answer is pretty simple: "When it stays put." Very soft collars or narrow ones will drive you crazy if you want them to stay outside your jacket, so don't bother.

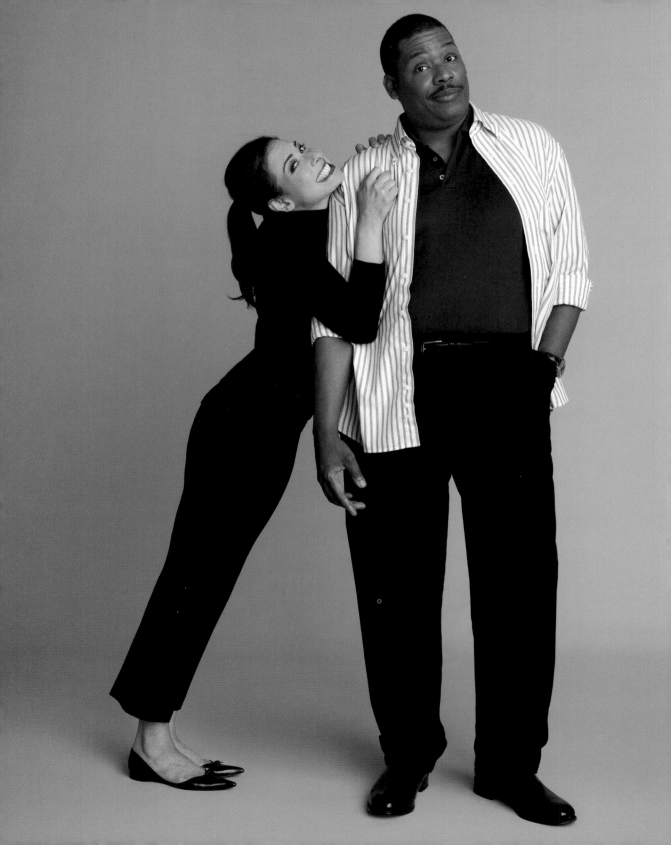

Hips
Weekend

As with suiting, most American-designer polo shirts are cut with extra room in the midsection, which makes them ideal for men with larger frames. When tucking in the shirt, blouse it a little at the waist.

Then top it with a button-front shirt. It's a perfect way to look casual and layered. The opening of the shirt also creates a strong vertical line down the front of the body, which is elongating and slimming.

When not wearing a jacket, go with a darker color trouser to reduce emphasis on the hip. And look for legs that remain wide through the length of the pant. You don't want to experience the ice-cream-cone effect, in which your legs resemble the shape of a cone, with your body as a scoop of Häagen-Dazs.

If you can, avoid pants with multiple pleats. It's difficult to find **flat** fronts in larger sizes, but keep the faith. If you must do a pleat, stick to a single one.

Universal Tip: Wearing flat-front pants? No need for a cuff.

Reality Check: Any time your body falls on the outer sides of the bell curve—either bigger or smaller than average—there lies the potential for shopping frustration. That's just the way it is; designers design to fit the most bodies possible, and some get lost in the process. That doesn't mean, however, that you should give up and wear sweatpants all the time. Talk to your tailor! If you carry your weight low on the body, you must, must, must fit the largest part of you and have the rest of the garment altered from there. Be sure your pants fit in the waist, hips, thighs, and butt. (You should have enough room to fit your hand comfortably into your waistband. Anything tighter will look uncomfortable and produce rolls where you don't want them.) If you find consequently that your pant legs are too wide, ask for them to be taken in a little down the line of the leg—without appearing too tapered.

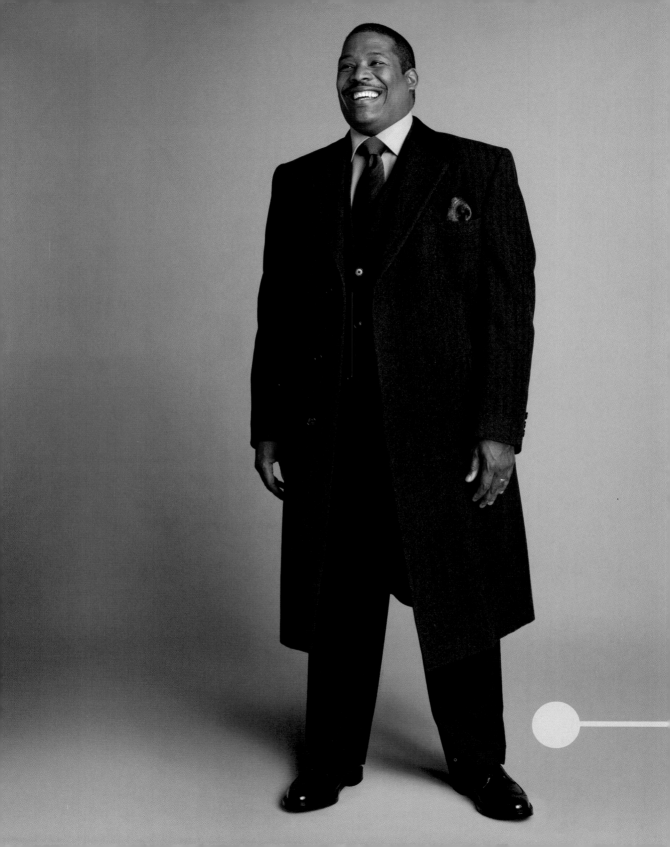

Hips

Evening

One look at Tony in this topcoat should have men running to their local specialty store. The topcoat is a wardrobe essential for dressy occasions: a wedding, a trip to the opera, a high-power business meeting. Buy the best one you can afford and think of it as an investment in style; not only will it never, ever go out of style, it forgives a multitude of sins. Even if your suit is off the sale rack, nobody would dare question it if you enter a room in a luxurious topcoat made of wool or cashmere or a blend of both.

When a man carries his weight on his lower half, the best way for him to balance out his body is to add a little bulk to his upper body. Here the strong-shouldered overcoat does the trick. The same effect could be achieved with a three-piece suit.

The length of the overcoat also works here because Tony's a tall man. If he were shorter, he could always have the coat shortened. A man's overcoat should never be floor length.

There are also several features bringing attention upward to the face: the brilliant color of the necktie, the pocket square, the contrasting velvet collar on the coat, the beautiful color of the shirt, and the large tie knot (because a big man needs a big knot in his tie).

Universal Tip: Men, reserve one pair of shiny black leather shoes for dressy occasions (we suggest two classics: a cap-toe laceup or a wing-tip). Don't wear them to work or for running errands on Sunday afternoon. A man's shoes tell a lot about who he is and how he takes care of himself. So when you're out on the town with the person you love, you'll want to look as put together and shined-up as possible. Who knows, you might even get lucky at the end of the night!

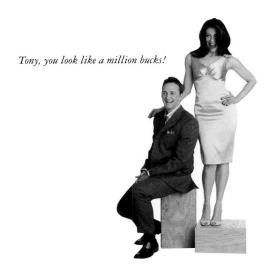

Tony, you look like a million bucks!

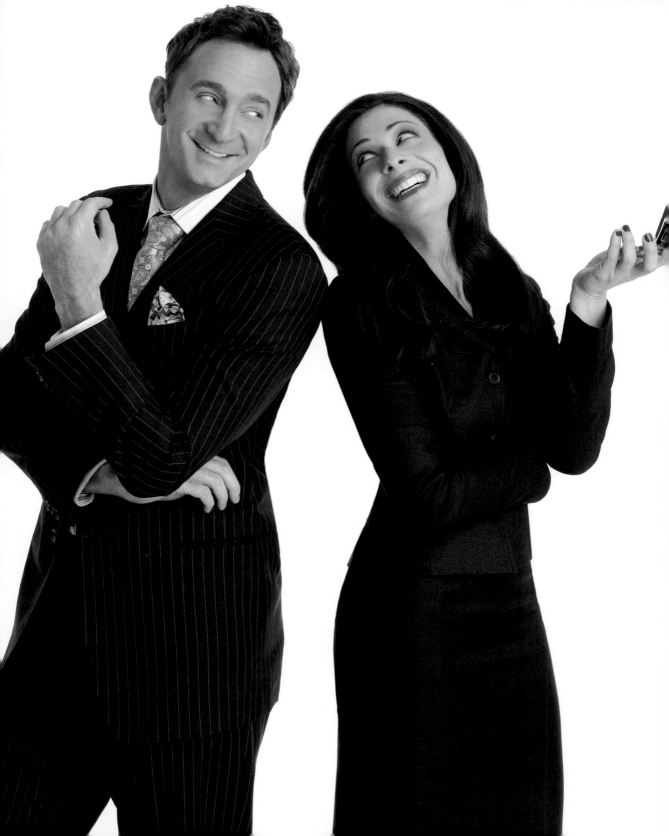

Afterword

Whew! We gotta tell ya, producing this book was a heck of a lot more work than either of us ever anticipated, but we're extremely proud of the final product. We can't thank our photographer, market editors, and hair and makeup team enough.

Most of all, however, we take our hats off to our models. Granted, it's pretty rare either of us wears a hat, as we're pretty particular about our hair, but still, in all seriousness, stripping down to a swimsuit in front of a camera is not a particularly enjoyable experience, especially when your photo could end up on a gazillion or so coffee tables. We all got through it together, though, with a lot of encouragement and a ton of laughs.

If you go back and look at any of the bathing suit photos, you'll have to imagine the two of us, somewhere off behind the camera yelling—above the din of the dance music—things like, "Shoulders back, big boobs out!" "Do it for hippy women everywhere!" and "Flex those muscles, you big stud!" And so, maybe you can think of us tomorrow morning while you're getting dressed whispering in your ear, "Love those thighs!" or "Work that tummy!" Honestly, we're all about making the best of what you've got. You really needn't have the "perfect" body to feel gorgeous and stylish.

And speaking of style, now that you have the basic tools, feel free to create a personal style all your own. Maybe you want to be the woman in your office known for her penchant for pointy-toed shoes or the guy who can sport a pocket square like no one's business. Hey, wait, that's our personal style! Go and get your own.

The Top Ten Questions We're Asked on an Almost-Daily Basis (Except There Are Only Eight of Them)

1. How do I look?

Accost us on the street and Stacy will be much more likely to answer that question honestly. Clinton, on the other hand, will usually say, "You look great," unless pressed for further explanation. Or offered money.

2. Where's Clinton/Stacy?

Contrary to popular belief, we don't spend all of our free time together, though it does seem like it sometimes. The way we figure it, based on the hours we have spent joined at the hip, we've spent as much time together as the average couple who's been married for five years.

SAYS CLINTON: "I have three stock answers for that question. One, 'She's in jail.' Two, 'She's locked in my basement.' And three, 'She's at home watching our kids.' I learned, however, that some people don't understand my sense of humor, so I'm less likely to use the one about the basement these days.

SAYS STACY: "I just say, 'He's not here, so stop looking around for him!'"

3. What did you do before this?

Stacy has been a fashion editor and stylist for, ummmm, a *lot* of years now. But she can't say how many because Clinton told her she should start lying about her age. Clinton was also a magazine editor for many years, and had a very short stint as a singing waiter in college.

4. Are you supposed to be wearing that?

Look, we run out of the house for milk, too. We go to the gym. Cut us some slack. We try to make sure that *most* of the time we are dressed our best, but no one's perfect.

5. When are you guys going to do a book?

Yeah, we know. It took us awhile. We've been busy. Here goes nothin'.

6. How did you two meet?

Our eyes locked across a crowded, smoky room and we knew we were destined to spend eternity together. (Actually, a casting director brought us together, but doesn't the other way sound more exciting?)

7. Do you style each other?

Not really. But we definitely value each other's opinion.

SAYS STACY: "Clinton doesn't usually say much of anything to me about my clothes, but when he really likes an outfit, he always says so. So basically he only likes about eighteen percent of my outfits."

CLINTON: "Sorry if I'm stingy with compliments. I just don't need your head getting any bigger than it already is."

8. Whose style do you admire the most?

SAYS STACY: "I've always been a massive fan of Kate Moss's style. She does it so effortlessly. But I also love the styles of the young Julie Christie, Jane Birkin, and Tuesday Weld. Lately Angelina Jolie has been rocking my world."

SAYS CLINTON: "I love the Old Hollywood look, à la Cary Grant, for dressier occasions. For casual wear, whoever styled Hugh Grant in *About a Boy* was a genius."

Acknowledgments

We would like to thank everyone who made this book possible—and that's a whole lot of people . . .

Lauren Galit, who fought to bring this project to life.

John Boswell, for keeping the dream alive.

Rick Horgan, for acquiring the project and for believing that we could meet our deadline, even if he did call us thirty times a day "just to check."

Dan Rembert, for stopping by the studio to watch and sending us cover mockups even though he didn't have to do either.

Elizabeth Van Itallie, Mark McCauslin, and **Linnea Knollmueller,** for turning the manuscript into a finished book.

Alonna Friedman, who simultaneously found our models *and* planned her wedding. If you were any more organized, you'd be a machine.

Christa Bourg, who took the helm of our project and steered it through to the bitter end. Bless you!

Brian Doben, our genius photographer whom we are now going to claim we discovered.

Nancy Corbett, who sat right behind Brian the whole time he was shooting and whispered gently in his ear when he left the lens cap on. We couldn't have asked for a better cheerleader.

Our models, for being brave in their bathing suits and beautiful inside and out.

Lee Harper, Eileen Goh, Jessica Neff, and **Kimberly Suggs,** who called in every stitch of clothing, all the shoes and accessories you saw, and about a hundred thousand other items you didn't see. You were tireless in your efforts and we thank you from the bottom of our hearts for all your hard work.

Regee Drummer (hair) and **Deanna Nickel** and **Matthew Nigara** (makeup). You are consummate artists who brought out the natural beauty of everyone in this book.

Steve Giralt, who showed us the true magic that is possible with digital photography.

Brad DeCecco, Masa Noguchi, and **Yoshi Suito,** who worked such long hours and never had anything but smiles on their faces . . . until our backs were turned.

Jeriana Hochberg, Garrett Munce, Deirdre Wegner, and **Lindsay "Ashley" Weiner,** who ran out and fetched different sizes in pants, skirts, shoes, and coffee cups and never charged anything extra on our credit cards. You were amazing to us.

Ania Jozwik, who made us the best food ever. We're still dreaming about the brownies!

Sara Jane Cohen, for accommodating us in every way possible and giving us a home for our backdrops.

Stacy would like to thank:

My family (Mommy, Nancy, Grandma, Poppyrazzi, Vickirazzi, and Babyrazzi), and all my friends, for inspiring me always and making me a better person every day I know them and for being so supportive even though they haven't actually seen me in person in three years.

Mark Riebling, who always said I should write something. And although he was probably thinking more along the lines of a "breakthrough" analysis of Aristotelian philosophy, he never failed to believe in me. Thank you, Bubuony.

Lisa Shotland, David Tenzer, and **Michael Yanover** at CAA for always taking my calls and giving me endless pep talks—and particularly to Lisa for always bringing on the booze at the right time.

A special thank-you to my **dad** and **stepmom,** who stopped by the studio to see what the hell the book was all about, eat a little food, and complain I would catch pneumonia in such a tiny dress.

And to **Clinton Kelly,** for putting up with me, laughing instead of crying, and for sharing in this amazing thing between us that everyone calls chemistry.

Clinton would like to thank:

The most amazingly supportive **family** anyone could ever ask for. I thank the Universe every day for putting *all* of you in my life.

Helen Shabason at ICM. For making me laugh and believing in me.

Jackie Eckhouse at Sloss Law. For reading the fine print.

Mr. Stiffler. For his incessant nagging—I mean, encouragement.

And **Stacy.** Oh, Stacy. How did this happen? One minute I'm putting my hand on your knee at an audition and the next we're inseparable. It's an absolute pleasure—99 percent of the time. I'd say 100 percent, but we'd both know I'd be lying. You're amazing.

Glossary

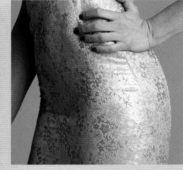

A-line: a skirt cut in the shape of a capital A. It's narrow at the waist and flares away from the hip.

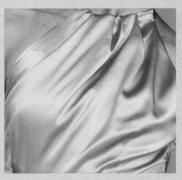

Brocade: a heavy fabric that's woven to produce a slightly raised (often floral) design.

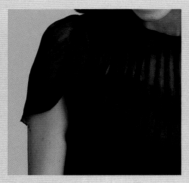

Charmeuse: a silk fabric with a satin (slightly glossy) finish.

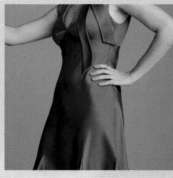

Bias cut: a term used when fabric is cut diagonally across the grain. The result is generally a garment that clings to your curves.

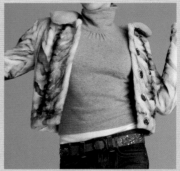

Cap sleeve: a little sleeve that covers the top shoulder.

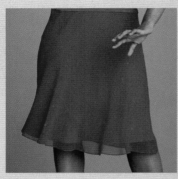

Chubby: a box jacket in a heavy fabric, leather, or fur.

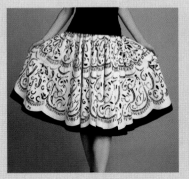

Circle skirt: a full skirt that's constructed by cutting a circle (or two halves of a circle) out of a piece of fabric.

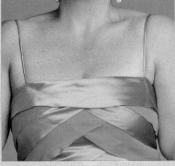

Décolleté: a low-cut neckline that reveals the shoulders and chest.

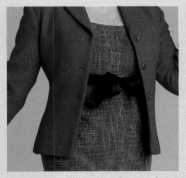

Empire seam, empire waist: a high-waisted seam that sits directly below the bustline.

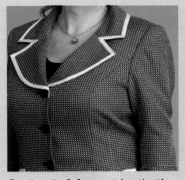

Contrast piping: a trim that's added along the seams of a garment or along the edges, as on a lapel.

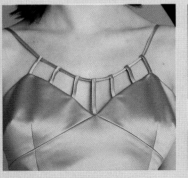

Dutchess satin: a satin that is heavier and stiffer than traditional satin.

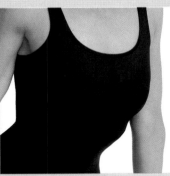

Girls, The: breasts, boobs, knockers, maracas, etc.

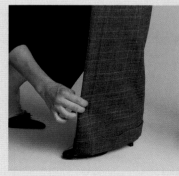

Glen plaid: a design that pairs small checks with larger checks in similar and often subdued colors.

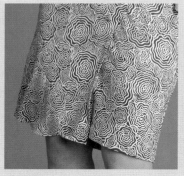

Jersey: fabric that is knitted in a plain stitch without a distinct rib.

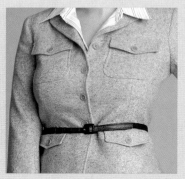

Lock and load (our term): keeping one's chest secured within a garment through the use of well-placed buttons.

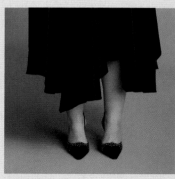

Handkerchief hem: the bottom of a dress or skirt cut to fall unevenly in points, at different lengths, alternately revealing or concealing leg.

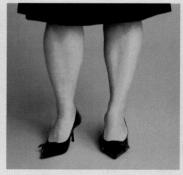

Kitten heel: a small, skinny heel, usually less than an inch. Also known as a Sabrina heel.

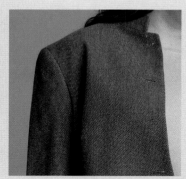

Nehru collar: a band of fabric at the neckline that stands up about an inch without the points of a traditional collar.

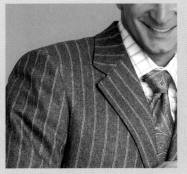

Notched lapel: a lapel with a V-shaped indentation.

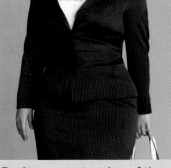

Peplum: an extension of the bodice of a dress or jacket that comes below the waistline, sometimes pleated or flared.

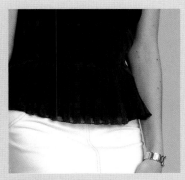

Pleating: a fold of fabric usually pressed flat but sometimes left unpressed. Vertical pleating. Inverse pleating.

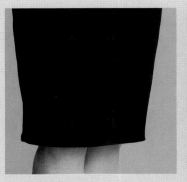

Pencil skirt: a straight skirt, which can narrow toward the hem or fall straight. It usually has a small back or side slit for ease of movement.

Placket pocket: a slit pocket without a covering flap.

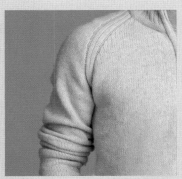

Raglan Sleeve: a sleeve that extends from the neckline, with a slanted seam from the neck to the underarm.

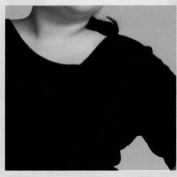

Rib: a corded effect in fabric that's created in the weaving process.

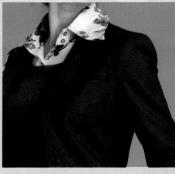

Schweaters (our term): sweaters with built-in (sometimes detachable) shirt collars and/or cuffs.

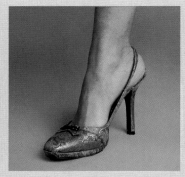

Sling-back: any shoe with an open back and a strap around the heel of the foot to hold it in place.

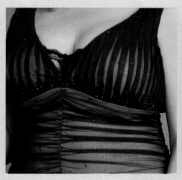

Ruching: fabric that's been gathered and stitched at a center point to maintain a rippled appearance.

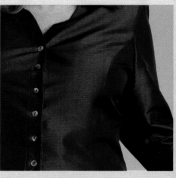

Shantung: a tightly woven fabric with twisted yarns that has the appearance of raw silk.

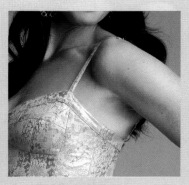

Spaghetti strap: a very thin strap that is sewn directly onto an otherwise strapless garment.

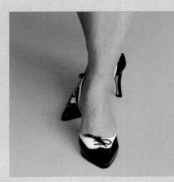

Spectator: a two-tone shoe frequently made in contrasting colors of black, navy, red, or brown on white or cream.

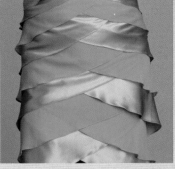

Tiers: layers of fabric placed one above another, sometimes on an angle.

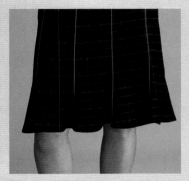

Trumpet skirt: a straight skirt with one large circular flounce at the hem that flares away from the body.

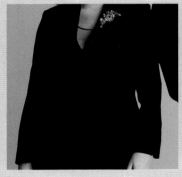

Stance: where the highest button on a jacket hits the chest. If the top button hits around the breastbone, it's considered a high stance; lower down on the abdomen, a low stance.

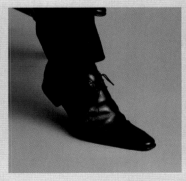

Toe box: the part of the shoe covering the toes that can be longer or shorter, depending on the design.

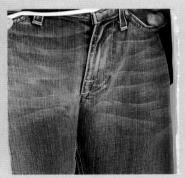

Whiskering: a distressing effect popular in denim that creates the look of worn-in creases on the hip and upper thigh.

Credits
WOMEN

Stacy
On Cover and Elsewhere: dress, Yigal Azrouel; earrings, Gerard Yosca; ring, Kenneth Jay Lane; shoes, Christian Louboutin
On Frontispiece and Elsewhere: dress, Dolce & Gabbana; shoes, Christian Louboutin; earrings, Gerard Yosca; ring, Kenneth Jay Lane
On Page 81 and Elsewhere: dress with lace inset, Anna Molinari; earrings, Gerard Yosca
On Page 103 and Elsewhere: dress, Moschino Cheap and Chic; shoes by Christian Louboutin; necklace, A. V. Max
On Page 236 and Elsewhere: suit, Dolce & Gabbana

Bigger on Top, Petite
Work: shirt, H&M; jacket and skirt, Anne Klein; shoes, Kors by Michael Kors.
Weekend: jeans, I.N.C.; jacket, Isabel & Nina; top, Karen Kane; shoes, BCBG Girls; bag, Maurizio Taiuti; necklace, RJ Graziano.
Evening: dress, Laundry; shoes, BCBG Girls; earrings, RJ Graziano.

Bigger on Top, Average Height
Work: dress, David Meister; turtleneck, Shin Choi; shoes, Juan Antonio Lopez from Searle; bag, Donald J. Pliner.
Weekend: shirt, Kulson; pants: How & Wen from Searle; shoes, Steven; jacket, Theory; bag: Talene Reilly.
Evening: dress, Nicole Miller Collection; shoes, Jean Michel Cazabat from Searle; pin, Monet; bracelet, R. J. Graziano.

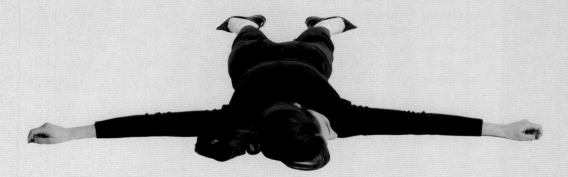

Bigger on Top, Tall

Work: top, Rafaella; jacket, Tahari; skirt, Tahari; earrings, Fragments; ring, Noir; shoes, N.Y.L.A.

Weekend: top, Ann Taylor; jacket, Liz Claiborne; skirt, Odille @ Anthropologie; earrings, Noir; bracelet/watch, Yochi & Lenni Navarro; shoes, Nancy Nancy.

Evening: dress, Dana Buchman; earrings, Fragments; bracelet/watch, Noir; scarf, Adrienne Landau; shoes, Ann Taylor.

Bigger on the Bottom, Petite

Work: cami, Anne Taylor Loft; jacket and skirt: Isabel & Nina; shoes, Franco Sarto; bag, Guess.

Weekend: jeans, Liz Claiborne; jacket, Andrew Marc; shirt, Shin Choi; shoes, Charles by Charles David.

Evening: dress, Ann Taylor; shoes, Michael Perry; pin, Ann Taylor; purse, Vintage Whiting & Davis; earrings: Vintage; pearls: RJ Graziano.

Bigger on the Bottom, Average Height

Work: shirt and jacket, Ann Klein; skirt, Nine West; shoes, Joan & David.

Weekend: shirt, Theory; jacket, Via Spiga; pants, Banana Republic; shoes, Charles Jourdan; bracelet, RJ Graziano, belt, Ellen Tracy; purple bag, Banana Republic.

Evening: dress, Laundry by Shelli Segal; shoes, Nine West; earrings and bracelets, RJ Graziano.

Bigger on the Bottom, Tall

Work: shirt, Lafayette 148; jacket, Lafayette 148; pants, AK Anne Klein; shoes, Nine West; watch, Anne Klein.

Weekend: shoes, Marc by Marc Jacobs; turtleneck, Shin Choi; skirt, H&M; bag, Nine West.

Evening: dress, David Meister; shoes, Aldo; earrings and bracelet, RJ Graziano.

A Little Extra in the Middle, Petite

Work: dress, Anne Klein; jacket, Lafayette 148; shoes, Christian Louboutin.

Weekend: jeans, Banana Republic; camisole, Only Hearts; jacket, Zara; bag, Adrienne Vittadini; necklace, Catherine Stein.

Evening: dress, Tadashi; shoes, Jill Stuart; scarf, Kenneth Cole; earrings, Robert Rose.

A Little Extra in the Middle, Average Height

Work: shirt, Kate Hill; suit, Cinzia Rocca; shoes, Cynthia Rowley; earrings, Liz Claiborne; watch, Anne Klein.

Weekend: jeans, Banana Republic; jacket, Nicole Miller; sweater, Jones New York Signature; shoes, Sacha London; earrings, Monet.

Evening: skirt, Due Per Due; blouse, Tadashi; shoes, Steve Madden; earrings, RJ Graziano.

A Little Extra in the Middle, Tall
Work: top, Rafaella; suit, Laura Biagiotti; brooch, Noir; bag, Pucci; shoes, Miu Miu.
Weekend: top, J. Crew; jacket, Mexx; pants, Banana Republic; necklaces, Fragments; scarf, Pucci; shoes, Joan & David.
Evening: jacket, Mexx; pants, Dolce & Gabbana; earrings, Yochi; rings, Noir; bag, Santi; shoes, Charles Jourdan.

Curvy, Petite
Work: camisole, Only Hearts; sweater, Laundry; shoes, Patrick Cox; bag, Coach; suit, Tadashi; necklace, Carolee.
Weekend: jeans, Banana Republic; blazer, Sud Express; shoes, BCBG; turtleneck, Cashmere 5th Avenue; bag, Banana Republic.
Evening: dress, Ruby Rox; shoes, Anne Klein; earrings, 2028.

Curvy, Average Height
Work: suit, Dolce & Gabbana; shoes, Christian Louboutin.
Weekend: top, DKNY; pants, Diesel; necklace, Wendy Mink; bag, leslie hsu; shoes, Valentino.
Evening: dress, Derek Lam; earrings, Noir NYC; shoes, Christian Louboutin; fur jacket, Jill Stuart.

Curvy, Tall
Work: jacket and skirt, Theory; blouse, Liquid; earrings, Sterling Silver; bag, Kenneth Cole; shoes, Charles Jourdan.
Weekend: dress, Diane Von Furstenberg; boots, Banana Republic; necklace, 2028.
Evening: dress, Tadashi; shoes, Martinez Valero; earrings, Monet; clutch, Banana Republic; bracelets, RJ Graziano.

Not Curvy, Petite
Work: top, Prada; shoes, Franco Sarto, with brooch by Liz Claiborne; earrings and watch, Cartier.
Weekend: shirt, Banana Republic; jacket, Zara; jeans, Fornarino; shoes, Franco Sarto; scarf, How & Wen.
Evening: dress, Miguelina; shoes, BCBG Max Azria; earrings, RJ Graziano.

Not Curvy, Average Height
Work: skirt and jacket, Nanette Lepore; camisole, Grassroots; shoes, Prada.
Weekend: shirt, Hugo Hugo Boss; jacket, Louie; pants, Zara; shoes, Nine West; necklace, RJ Graziano.
Evening: dress, David Meister; shoes, Nine West; bag, Donald J. Pliner; earrings, RJ Graziano.

Not Curvy, Tall

Work: pants, Anne Klein; shirt, Anne Klein; vest, Parronchi from Searle; shoes, Linda Allard for Ellen Tracy.

Weekend: sweater, Shin Choi; tank, J. Crew; jeans, Notify; boots, Ellen Tracy; coat, Dana Buchman; belt, Chan Luu.

Evening: skirt, Monica from Searle; top, Shin Choi; shoes, BCBG Girls; necklace, RJ Graziano; bracelet, Monet.

Extra Curvy, Petite

Work: jacket, Richard Metzger; shirt, Krazy Kat; skirt, Richard Metzger; shoes, Samanth· Shoes; necklace, stylists' own

Weekend: jeans, Lane Bryant Seven; jacket, Lafayette 148; sweater, Kirkland Signature; boots, Via Spiga; bag, Kenneth Cole.

Evening: camisole, Lane Bryant; skirt, Richard Metzger; shawl, Kenneth Cole; earrings and shoes, model's own.

Extra Curvy, Average Height

Work: top and skirt, Lafayette 148; shoes, Charles Jourdan; bag, Chanel; earrings, Charter Club; bracelet, stylists' own.

Weekend: shirt, Lafayette 148; jeans, Mossimo from Target; earrings, Liz Claiborne.

Evening: shoes, Samanth Shoes; dress, Niki Livas; earrings, RJ Graziano; clutch, stylists' own.

Extra Curvy, Tall

Work: top, pants and jacket, Lafayette 148; shoes, Parade; necklace, stylists' own.

Weekend: top and pants, Lane Bryant; boots, Samanth Shoes; earrings, RJ Graziano.

Evening: shirt, Essendi; skirt, Lane Bryant; shoes, Samanth Shoes; jewelry: stylists' own.

MEN

Clinton

On Cover and Elsewhere: suit, Paul Smith; shirt, Sean John; pocket square, City of London; belt, Banana Republic; shoes Bally

On Frontispiece and Elsewhere: suit, Corneliani; shirt, BCBG; pocket square, Pucci; belt, Cole Haan; shoes, Bruno Magli

On page 236: suit, Giorgio Armani; shirt, Paul Smith; tie, Richard James; pocket square, Pucci

Short

Work: shirt, DKNY; overcoat, Hugo Boss; pants, J. Crew; belt, Banana Republic; shoes, Lambertson Truex.

Weekend: jacket, Diesel; shirt, Kenneth Cole; pants, Diesel; shoes, Puma.

Evening: suit, Gieves; shirt, Zegna; tie, Giorgio Armani; belt, Coach; shoes, Cole Haan.

Average

Work: suit, Ted Baker; shirt, Gant; shoes, Ted Baker; tie, Ted Baker; belt, Allen Edmonds from Zappos.com; pocket square, Jay Kos.

Weekend: T-shirt, Polo Ralph Lauren; pants, Polo Ralph Lauren; sweater, Gant; jacket, Paul Stuart; shoes, Vigotti from Zappos.com; umbrella, Barney's New York.

Evening: suit, Ted Baker; shirt, Robert Graham; belt, Allen Edmonds from Zappos.com; pocket square, Jay Kos; shoes, Vigotti from Zappos.com.

Tall

Work: suit, Lanvin; shirt, Paul Smith; tie, Robert Talbott; belt, Cole Haan; pocket square, Robert Talbott; shoes, Cole Haan.

Weekend: cardigan, Marc Jacobs; T-shirt, John Varvatos; pants, G-Star; shoes, Asics.

Evening: jacket, Ted Baker; shirt, Michael Kors; pants, Calvin Klein; belt, Coach; shoes, Jean-Baptiste Rautureau.

Athletic

Work: shirt, Etro; pants, Jay Kos; jacket, Jay Kos; shoes, Type Z; belt, Gant.

Weekend: sweater, I.N.C.; pants, Jay Kos; shoes, Ted Baker; bag, Ben Sherman; watch, TAG Heuer Monoco.

Evening: shirt, Ted Baker; jeans, Ted Baker Jean; belt, Gant; shoes, Donald J. Pliner; jacket, DKNY.

Small-Framed

Work: tie, Etro; shirt, Agnès B.; suit, Emporio Armani; shoes, Ferragamo; belt, Cole Haan; watch, Emporio Armani; pocket square, Jay Kos.

Weekend: T-Shirt, Fruit of the Loom from Urban Outfitters; pants, H&M; sweater, H&M; boots, Ferragamo.
Evening: pants, Etro; sweater, Etro; jacket, Bill Tornade; sneakers, Puma.

Barrel-Chested

Work: shirt, Jay Kos; pants, Jay Kos; jacket, Jay Kos; shoes, Vigotti from Zappos.com; briefcase, Hartmann; watch, TAG Heuer.
Weekend: sweater, Gant; pants, Nautica; shoes, Timberland; T-shirt, Polo Ralph Lauren; sunglasses, Fendi.
Evening: jeans, Ted Baker Jean; shirt, Jay Kos; tie, Ted Baker; jacket, Ted Baker; shoes, Type Z; belt, Etro.

Tummy

Work: sweater, Kenneth Cole; pants, Dockers; shoes, Polo Ralph Lauren; jacket, Kasper.
Weekend: sweater, Joseph Abboud; pants, Polo Ralph Lauren; shoes, Clarks; jacket, Boss Hugo Boss; scarf, Gant.
Evening: jeans, Robert Graham; shoes, Bruno Magli; shirt, Robert Graham; jacket, Gant.

Hips

Work: pants, George Foreman Signature Collection; sweater, Nat Nast; coat, Tommy Hilfiger; shoes, Bruno Magli from Zappos.com; briefcase, Gant.
Weekend: polo shirt, Ralph Lauren; button-front shirt, Gant; pants, George Foreman; shoes, Florsheim from Zappos.com; watch: TAG Heuer—the Steve McQueen; belt, Allen Edmonds from Zappos.com.
Evening: suit, Calvin Klein; shirt, Gant; shoes, Florsheim from Zappos.com; belt, Allen Edmonds from Zappos.com; tie, Jay Kos; pocket square, Ruffian; overcoat, Petrocelli.

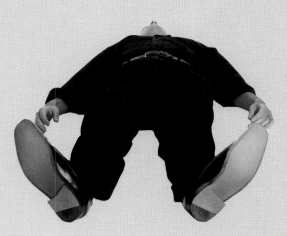

About the Authors

Each week millions of viewers tune in to see whether **Clinton Kelly**, cohost of TLC's *What Not to Wear,* can successfully transform yet another fashion eyesore into an aesthetically pleasing member of society. With his trademark combination of good-natured humor, honest observation, and expert styling advice, Clinton helps men and women of all ages, shapes, and sizes refine their appearance, increase their self-esteem, and kick-start goals into reality.

Before joining *What Not to Wear,* Clinton held the position of executive editor at *DNR,* the well-respected menswear fashion and news weekly trade magazine. Prior to that, he was the deputy editor of *Mademoiselle,* where, among other responsibilities, he penned an advice column under the pseudonym Joe L'Amour. He was also a contributing editor to *Marie Claire,* where he oversaw dozens of stories on beauty and clothing. In the early '90s, Clinton was a host of *Q2,* an experimental television channel launched for QVC by Barry Diller.

Clinton was raised in Port Jefferson Station, Long Island. He received his B.A. in communications from Boston College and his master's degree in journalism from Northwestern University. His turn-ons include mosaics, most cheeses, and Olivia Newton-John. His turn-offs include the musical *Cats,* ingrown hairs, and people who say things like "I'm a really complex individual."

As the original cohost of *What Not to Wear,* **Stacy London** has spent the last three years sharing her knowledge of high fashion and styling expertise with the fashionably challenged, attempting to help unlock the inner-style diva in all of us.

Stacy brings with her to the show fifteen years of styling experience. After graduating Phi Beta Kappa from Vassar College with a double degree in twentieth-century philosophy and German literature, she began her career at *Vogue* magazine as a fashion assistant and later returned to Condé Nast as the senior fashion editor at *Mademoiselle.* She has styled fashion photos for such editorial publications as *Italian D, Nylon,* and *Contents.*

Stacy has worked with numerous celebrities and fashion shows. Over the last three years, she has also worked with a diverse group of advertising clients such as Wonderbra, Proctor and Gamble, Covergirl, Target, Levi's, Maytag, Bali, Swatch USA, Longines, and, most recently, Calvin Klein. She has appeared on many national talk shows, including *Oprah, Today, Weekend Today,* CNN, *The Jane Pauley Show, The Early Show,* and Showtime's *American Candidate.*

A native of Manhattan, Stacy now resides in Brooklyn with her two fabulously fashionable cats, Moo and Al, and many, many pairs of stilettos.

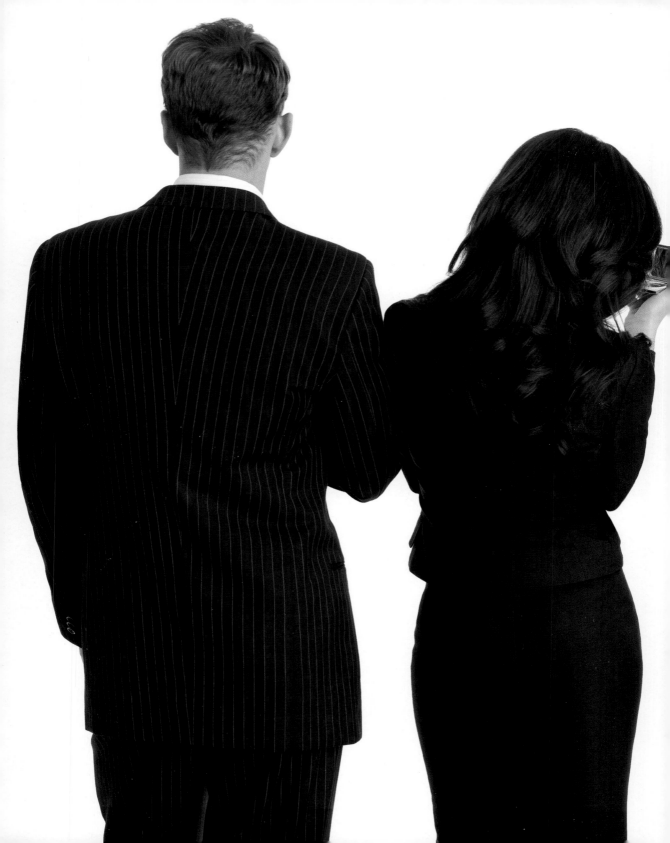